Camberwell Assessment of Need: Forensic Version

2nd edition

Camberwell Assessment of Need: Forensic Version

2nd edition

CANFOR

Stuart Thomas
RMIT University

Mike Slade
University of Nottingham

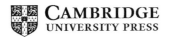
CAMBRIDGE
UNIVERSITY PRESS

CAMBRIDGE
UNIVERSITY PRESS

University Printing House, Cambridge CB2 8BS, United Kingdom

One Liberty Plaza, 20th Floor, New York, NY 10006, USA

477 Williamstown Road, Port Melbourne, VIC 3207, Australia

314–321, 3rd Floor, Plot 3, Splendor Forum, Jasola District Centre,
New Delhi – 110025, India

79 Anson Road, #06–04/06, Singapore 079906

Cambridge University Press is part of the University of Cambridge.
It furthers the University's mission by disseminating knowledge in the pursuit of
education, learning, and research at the highest international levels of excellence.

www.cambridge.org
Information on this title: www.cambridge.org/9781911623410
DOI: 10.1017/9781911623427

First published 2003, Gaskell, The Royal College of Psychiatrists
This second edition published by Cambridge University Press 2021

Printed in the United Kingdom by TJ Books Limited, Padstow Cornwall

A catalogue record for this publication is available from the British Library.

ISBN 978-1-911-62341-0 Paperback

Contents

Acknowledgements

The authors would like to express thanks to the following people who contributed to the development of the CANFOR scales and publication of the original CANFOR book, published by the Royal College of Psychiatrists in 2003: Paul McCrone, Janet Parrott, Mari-Anne Harty, and Graham Thornicroft.

We would also like to acknowledge John Basson, Pamela Taylor, Martin Butwell, Tim Green, James Noak, Lisa Davies, Morven Leese, and the many other staff and service users who made the development of the CANFOR scales possible.

Abbreviations

CAN	Camberwell Assessment of Need
CANDID	Camberwell Assessment of Need for Adults with Developmental and Intellectual Disabilities
CANE	Camberwell Assessment of Need for the Elderly
CANFOR	Camberwell Assessment of Need Forensic Version (including CANFOR-S, CANFOR-R, and CANFOR-C)
CANFOR-C	Camberwell Assessment of Need Forensic Clinical Version
CANFOR-R	Camberwell Assessment of Need Forensic Research Version
CANFOR-S	Camberwell Assessment of Need Forensic Short Version
HESPER	Humanitarian Emergency Settings Perceived Needs Scale
HoNOS	Health of the Nation Outcome Scale
MDO	Mentally disordered offender
NHS	National Health Service
PRiSM	The Psychiatric Research in Service Measurement team, which was in the Section of Community Psychiatry at the Institute of Psychiatry, London
SMI	Severe mental illness

Introduction

The Camberwell Assessment of Need Forensic Version (CANFOR) is an individual needs assessment scale designed to identify the needs of people with mental health concerns who are in contact with forensic mental health services. It was developed by members of the Section of Community Psychiatry at the Institute of Psychiatry in London, in collaboration with clinicians at the Bracton Centre, a secure psychiatric facility operated by Oxleas NHS Foundation Trust. The CANFOR is based on the Camberwell Assessment of Need (CAN), a needs assessment scale designed to assess the needs of people with severe and/or enduring mental health problems (Phelan et al., 1995; Slade et al., 1999; Slade & Thornicroft, 2020).

The CANFOR covers a broad range of health, social, clinical, and functional needs and ensures that the common needs of forensic mental health service users will be assessed. Different viewpoints are recorded separately in the scales; this allows for staff, service user, and carer views to be considered and documented alongside each other in one complete assessment. A complete assessment therefore serves to highlight both agreement and disagreement in perceptions of need between different people and is intended to form the basis of further discussions aimed at devising the optimum care and treatment planning for the individual.

This is the 2nd edition of the CANFOR book; the 1st edition was published by the Royal College of Psychiatrists in 2003. In this 2nd edition, we provide some updated guidance and minor changes, reflecting on our experiences with its implementation and use for research and in routine clinical practice over the last 18 years. Of specific note, we have changed the name and scope of two of the CANFOR domains to better reflect contemporary situations and circumstances. We have changed the Child Care domain to Dependents in this 2nd edition, to reflect changes that are emerging associated with an ageing population.

We have also changed the Telephone domain to Digital Communication to better reflect other additional and/or alternative ways of communicating with others (for example, through social media). We have also changed how the need rating for each of the 25 CANFOR domains is recorded in all variants of the CANFOR scales. In the 1st edition, we used a numeric scoring system (where 0 = no need, 1 = met need, 2 = unmet need, 8 = not applicable, and 9 = not known in the need domain). In this 2nd edition, we have changed the rating to use letters ('N' for no need, 'M' for met need, 'U' for unmet need, 'NA' for not applicable, and '?' for not known) instead of numbers. These changes reflect those made to the 2nd edition of the Camberwell Assessment of Need (Slade & Thornicroft, 2020).

The CANFOR is administered as a semi-structured interview to screen for identifiable areas of need, but it does not assess identified problems in detail. Therefore, needs that are identified through the assessment process may require further investigation and assessment using appropriate standardised scales (for example, psychological distress, safety to self, safety to others, sexual offences, and arson).

Three versions of the CANFOR have been developed, each covering the same 25 domains of need. Comprehensive versions are available for research use (CANFOR-R), and clinical use (CANFOR-C). They identify the presence of a need and record the level of help received from different sources (both from informal sources such as friends and family and from formal sources such as statutory services). They also identify the person's overall satisfaction with the help they have received from services and consider, from the staff member's perspective, whether difficulties in specific areas may have contributed to the index offence or reason for referral to the service. A short summary version of CANFOR is also available (CANFOR-S), which simply records the presence of a need (i.e. the need rating) in each of the 25 domains of need and whether that need is 'met' or 'unmet' by considering any help currently being received. The CANFOR-S is suitable for both research and clinical use; we have found that it also tends to be the CANFOR scale of choice, both for research and in routine clinical practice.

This book provides the necessary information so that the CANFOR scales can be used without the need for formal training. Chapter 2 provides a brief overview of needs assessment and a discussion of specific issues relating to people who receive support and care from forensic mental health services. Chapter 3 describes the development of the CANFOR scales. Chapter 4 contains descriptions of the 25 need domains (including changes from the 1st edition of the book and scales). Chapter 5 provides guidance for using the full research version (CANFOR-R), and Chapter 6 provides guidance for the full clinical version (CANFOR-C). Chapter 7 focuses on the short version of the assessment (CANFOR-S) and provides instructions

for its use. Chapter 8 provides some details on translations of the CANFOR scales that have been completed and brief details about those that have been published. Chapter 9 suggests a structure for a training session that can be delivered in house to help familiarise appropriate staff and researchers with the CANFOR scales and how to complete them. It includes three short vignettes and one full vignette so that readers can practice the completion of the scales. Chapter 10 includes a number of frequently asked questions, and Chapter 11 provides a comprehensive list of references. A series of appendices are also included. Appendices 1, 2, and 3 provide copies of the three CANFOR scales. Appendix 4 provides copies of suggested summary score sheets for the CANFOR-R and CANFOR-C. These appendices are provided in a format that is suitable for scanning and can be freely photocopied. The fifth and final appendix provides a copy of the original psychometric evaluation of the CANFOR, published in 2008.

Needs Assessment

Needs assessment has long been a required component of mental health services planning, development, and evaluation and continues to play a central role in contemporary mental health policy. In order to understand needs assessment, its role in the commissioning of services, and recommendations that it is used in routine clinical practice, it is first necessary to define the terminology that is involved, then examine ways in which needs have been assessed in mental health services. Consideration of additional factors regarding the care and treatment of forensic mental health service users is then also required.

2.1 Need in Relation to Mental Health Services

Various definitions of need have been offered since the UK-based National Health Service and Community Care Act 1990 (Department of Health, 1991) made the recommendation that care and treatment should be based on assessments of individual need. These definitions have included issues related to quality of life, restoring and maintaining suitable levels of independence, and the ability to benefit from health care (NHS Management Executive, 1990; Stevens & Gabbay, 1991). Broadly speaking, two approaches to assessing needs were developed: normative approaches and subjective approaches. The normative approach stipulated that needs should be assessed by professionals and that needs are only identified where problems are remediable through intervention. The CANFOR, by contrast, is based on the second approach – a subjective model of need, which recognises that different yet equally valid views of need can and do exist.

At the time of publishing the first edition of this book, this approach of increased service-user involvement in forensic mental health services was considered innovative. There was incontrovertible evidence, emanating from general mental health service reforms,

that showed that service-user views of their needs should be taken into account in all aspects of mental health care and treatment planning, especially in instances where disagreements are evident between staff and service-user perspectives (Slade, 1996; Slade, 1998). Indeed, for more than 20 years, it has been argued that the views of service users are the most important (Department of Health, 1999). While these developments progressed relatively quickly in the general mental health sector, such reforms were slower to emerge in forensic mental health services. It became increasingly apparent that while the needs of forensic service users were similar to those in other mental health services, they were also characteristically different in other ways, and that this therefore potentially warranted additional consideration.

Arguably one of the key catalysts for change in forensic mental health was the publication of a significant report on the care and treatment of mentally disordered offenders, known as The Reed Report, published by the Department of Health and Home Office in 1992. The Reed Report sought to review what health and social services were available for mentally disordered offenders and determine whether current services needed to change – and, if so, how these changes could be implemented. It followed earlier reports, most notably the Glancy Report and Butler Reports, and recommendations from the UK-based Royal College of Psychiatrists, which all emphasized the need for a range of secure services to be available for the care and treatment of mentally disordered offenders. The Reed Report noted that care and treatment of mentally disordered offenders often fell far short of what was needed or indeed considered desirable. Further, it recommended that care and treatment should be provided by health and social services, because the needs of mentally disordered offenders were identified as being primarily medical and social in focus (Chiswick, 1992). Importantly here, the Reed Report also emphasized that care should be provided on the basis of individual need. The assessment of need was central here because levels of security were to be defined by the type and extent of needs presented by the service user (Chiswick, 1992; Isweran & Bardsley, 1987).

After the publication of an article by Shaw (2002), which reiterated that forensic patients are different and therefore that their needs will be different, an evidence base about the nature and extent of the individual needs of forensic mental health service users started to be developed and gradually disseminated. Indeed, the first edition of the CANFOR book was published in the following year (Thomas et al., 2003). Of note here, this increased interest also led to the Health of the National Outcome Scale (HoNOS) being adapted and a new HoNOS-secure tool being proposed (Dickens, Sugarman & Walker, 2007) – although it retained the clinical only rated assessment, thus missing out on clearly discernible differences in (equally, if not more valid) perceptions of need.

Since the publication of the first edition of the CANFOR book, assessments of the individual needs of forensic mental health service users have been reported across the international literature. These developments were spearheaded, in part, by the publication of a series of articles based on a project that sought to define the individual and placement needs of inpatients across the three high-security psychiatric hospitals in the UK. These studies were important in terms of developing the evidence base around the needs of forensic mental health service users, demonstrating pertinent differences in needs between patients requiring different levels of security (Harty et al., 2004; Thomas, Dolan, & Thornicroft, 2004; Thomas et al., 2004), as well as differences between females and males, along with differences in perceptions of need between staff members and service users. Further publications have separately detailed the need of different groups in high-security psychiatric services, including women (Thomas et al., 2005), people detained under the legal category of psychopathic disorder (Dolan et al., 2005), and people with intellectual disabilities (Thomas et al., 2004). Using the CANFOR in these and a series of subsequent studies has helped inform service reform initiatives and the development of more specialist service responses for different special needs populations who are cared for and treated in secure psychiatric settings.

2.2 Research Applications of and Findings Using the CANFOR

International research has now reported levels and common profiles of need across the full range of forensic mental health services. While there has inevitably been a degree of variability between individual study findings, due to a range of methodological and sampling issues, some general patterns have emerged in relation to the total number of needs and the proportion of these that are rated as being unmet.

An interesting recent example of how need profiles differ by level of security is found in an Australian study reported by Adams and colleagues (2018). Their study profiled a full cohort of forensic mental health service users in the State of New South Wales, reporting staff ratings of the needs of service users in prison, high-security, medium-security, low-security, open security, and community settings. It should be noted here that definitions of different levels of security may vary according to jurisdiction (e.g., Adams et al., 2019). The general trend is that as the level of security reduces, so does the total number of needs reported. The same pattern emerges with consideration of unmet needs, with decreasing numbers of unmet needs as the level of security of the service decreases. Prison-based research using the CANFOR has reported much higher proportions of unmet needs, both from staff and service-user perspectives (e.g. Harty et al., 2012; Shepherd, Ogloff, & Thomas, 2016; Thomas, McCrone, & Fahy, 2009). The Adams et al. (2018) study suggests that community forensic mental health users have total need and unmet need profiles similar to those people being treated in medium-security services.

International research has also reported that while staff and service-user assessments of individual needs have a good deal of overlap, they do differ in several key (and important) aspects. Again, this body of research reinforces the need to assess both staff and service user perceptions of need separately in a single assessment.

2.3 Application of the CANFOR in Clinical Practice

The CANFOR has been found feasible for use in clinical practice, with Long and colleagues (2008) reporting that the results of CANFOR assessments were perceived as useful by both staff and service users. Published translations of the CANFOR have also concluded that the scales have clinical utility (Castelletti et al., 2015; Romeva et al., 2010; Talina et al., 2013).

A recent Australian study that considered the applicability of a range of routine outcome measures being used in forensic mental health services reported that while the nationally mandated general mental health measures (the Health of the National Outcome Scale (HoNOS) and Life Skills Profile (LSP-16)) had some utility, they lacked important treatment planning information specific to forensic environments (Shinkfield & Ogloff, 2014). In a subsequent publication, the authors recommended the CANFOR as one of six routine outcome measures suitable for use in forensic mental health services (Shinkfield & Ogloff, 2015).

2.4 Broader Considerations

Livingston, Rossiter, and Verdun-Jones (2011) have cautioned about the potential negative connotations of the forensic label, noting that while the term may be used administratively to denote that a person is being treated by forensic services (e.g. Buchanan & Wootton, 2002), this can lead to much more pejorative labels, commonly associated with dangerousness and criminality. Hartwell (2004) suggested that this combination (adding substance misuse to the challenges of having received a mental illness diagnosis and having a criminal history) can lead to a 'triple stigma' and thus further compound people's chances of successful community reintegration.

Barnao and Ward (2015) posit that one of the key challenges facing modern-day forensic mental health services is that they are operating from two quite different paradigms – a psychopathology paradigm and a risk assessment and management paradigm – with different purposes and functions (one of care and one of custody). Given these additional risks of social marginalisation and the challenges of community reintegration, it is arguably all the more important to consider and centrally include the needs of forensic mental health service users in all aspects of their care, treatment, and rehabilitation.

More recently published research has considered the interface and interconnections between the constructs of need, risk, and recovery. While any detailed discussion extends beyond the current text, this research has demonstrated how need, as assessed by the CANFOR, is correlated with established measures of risk and recovery. For example, the recent Australian study referred to previously (Adams et al., 2018) reported that higher total needs were associated with greater risk, as assessed using the HCR-20 (Douglas et al., 2013), and lower rates of treatment completion and recovery, as assessed using the DUNDRUM-3 and DUNDRUM-4 (Kennedy et al., 2010). These research findings, along with others (e.g. Abou-Sinna & Luebbers, 2012), are very positive and indicate that the CANFOR fills an important role, value adding to core measures of risk and recovery that are central to forensic mental health services delivery. As Davoren and colleagues (2012) note, this fuller picture allows clinicians and service planners to more fully consider the past severity of behaviours, while also better considering measures of progress for individual service users.

Development of the Camberwell Assessment of Need Forensic Version (CANFOR)

The CANFOR is an assessment that highlights a range of problem areas that people in contact with forensic mental health services may experience and/or present to services with. It was developed for use across the full range of forensic mental health services, including high-, medium-, and low-security psychiatric services; community forensic mental health services; probation services; and prison services. The basic premise behind this is that it provides a consistent means of assessing needs and therefore a consistent language that can be used across all levels and types of forensic services. An added advantage is that profiles of need (total number of needs, number of unmet needs, and number of met needs) can be measured and directly compared across service groupings.

The contents and structure of the CANFOR scales are based on the adult Camberwell Assessment of Need (CAN), which was developed by staff at the Section of Community Psychiatry (PRiSM) team at the Institute of Psychiatry in London (Phelan et al., 1995; Slade et al., 1999; Slade & Thornicroft, 2020). The CANFOR was developed by members of the same team, in collaboration with clinicians working in forensic mental health services in Oxleas NHS Foundation Trust.

The validity and reliability of CANFOR were initially investigated in medium- and high-security psychiatric hospitals, with an article describing its psychometric properties published in the *International Journal of Methods in Psychiatric Research* in 2008 (Thomas et al., 2008; see Appendix 5). The CANFOR has since been used for research purposes and in clinical settings across the full range of forensic mental health services and across multiple countries. The CANFOR has also been independently recommended as a routine outcome measure for use in forensic mental health services (Shinkfield & Ogloff, 2014; Shinkfield & Ogloff, 2015).

The adult CAN was developed as an assessment measure to identify the health and social needs of adults of working age with mental health problems. Details of the psychometric properties of the CAN

assessment were originally provided in an article by Phelan et al. (1995). As the adult CAN was not intended for use in all areas of mental health services, a number of variants have been developed for use with other populations, including the following:

- Camberwell Assessment of Need – Elderly (CANE), which assesses the needs of adults over the age of 65 years (Reynolds et al., 2000)
- Camberwell Assessment of Need – Developmental and Intellectual Disabilities (CANDID), which assesses the needs of adults with learning disabilities and mental health problems (Xenitidis et al., 2000)
- Camberwell Assessment of Need – Mothers (CAN-M), which assesses the needs of pregnant women and mothers with severe mental illness (Howard et al., 2008)
- Camberwell Assessment of Need Forensic Version (CANFOR), which assesses the needs of people in contact with forensic mental health services (Thomas et al., 2003; Thomas et al., 2008)
- Humanitarian Emergency Settings Perceived Needs (HESPER) scale (Semrau et al., 2012), for people in disaster relief situations

CAN variants have since been used extensively in both research and clinical settings and have been translated into a number of other languages. There is an overlap between each of the CAN variants, with 'core' health and social needs common to all CAN variants and needs specific to each population also included. All variants of the CAN have been developed according to the same principles, and they assess need in exactly the same way: The four underlying principles (from Johnson et al., 1996) are as follows:

1. Needs are universal;
2. Many psychiatric patients have multiple needs;
3. Needs assessment should be a routine part of clinical practice; and
4. The needs assessment process should include ratings by both staff and patients.

The CAN was developed according to the following criteria:

1. That it would have adequate psychometric properties;
2. That it could be completed in 30 minutes or less;
3. That it would be comprehensive;
4. That is measured both met and unmet need;
5. That it would be useable by a wide range of mental health professionals;
6. That it could record help received from friends or relatives, as well as from statutory services, and that these are recorded separately; and
7. That it would be suitable for use in research and in routine clinical practice.

Three versions of the CANFOR have been developed using these criteria, and those described by Salvador-Carulla (1996) and are available for research or clinical use. These are:

- CANFOR-R – a comprehensive research version (see Chapter 5 and Appendix 1)
- CANFOR-C – a comprehensive clinical version (see Chapter 6 and Appendix 2)
- CANFOR-S – a brief one-page version for research or routine clinical use (see Chapter 7 and Appendix 3)

A number of queries about the development and use of the CANFOR are addressed in Chapter 10 (Frequently Asked Questions). Many of these are common to all CAN variants. If you find that answers to your questions are not sufficiently addressed in this book, then consult additional resources available through the Research into Recovery website (http://researchintorecovery.com/can) or contact the lead author of the CANFOR, Professor Stuart Thomas.

3.1 Psychometric Properties of the CANFOR

An article describing the psychometric properties of the CANFOR was published in 2008 in the *International Journal of Methods in Psychiatric Research* (Thomas et al., 2008). A full copy of this article is provided in Appendix 5. In brief, content validity was sought from a sample of inpatients in medium- and high-security psychiatric services in two services in Southern England, and consensual validity was considered by surveying a group of fifty forensic mental health professionals across the United Kingdom. Face validity and construct validity were also explored; all were considered appropriate. Inter-rater reliability (i.e. the extent to which two or more raters agree) and test-retest reliability (i.e. how consistent ratings are over time) were also calculated; inter-rater reliability was reported as 0.991 for service-user ratings and 0.998 for staff ratings; test-retest reliability was 0.795 for service-user ratings and 0.852 for staff ratings; these were considered adequate.

Similar reliability and validity results have been reported with the Spanish, Portuguese, and Italian translations of the CANFOR. Collectively, these studies suggest that the CANFOR is a valid and reliable measure that is suited for routine clinical use and that has utility in practice.

Practicalities of Using the CANFOR Scales

All three CANFOR variants assess the same 25 domains of need:

1. Accommodation
2. Food
3. Looking after the Living Environment
4. Self-Care
5. Daytime Activities
6. Physical Health
7. Psychotic Symptoms
8. Information about Condition and Treatment
9. Psychological Distress
10. Safety to Self
11. Safety to Others
12. Alcohol
13. Drugs
14. Company
15. Intimate Relationships
16. Sexual Expression
17. Dependents
18. Basic Education
19. Digital Communication
20. Transport
21. Money
22. Budgeting
23. Treatment
24. Sexual Offending
25. Arson

Note changes from the 1st edition include renaming two of the need domain names – Dependents and Digital Communication. In the 1st edition, Dependents was named 'Child Care'. Consistent with the Camberwell Assessment of Need (CAN), 2nd edition (Slade & Thornicroft, 2020), we have changed the domain name to Dependents to better reflect changes associated with an ageing population. Additionally, the 1st edition need domain entitled 'Telephone' has been renamed Digital Communication to better capture the increased

number of ways we can communicate with other people (for example, with social media).

Opening prompt (trigger) questions are provided to start the conversation on a particular topic area. A mixture of open and closed questions should then be used, with the aim of establishing if the person has had any problems/difficulties in the particular domain during the last month. If any problems/difficulties are identified, the interviewer should then go on to explore whether the person has been receiving any help for this particular problem/difficulty in the last month, both formally from services and informally through friends and family, and if so, whether this help has been effective or not.

Of note, the scoring of each need domain is based directly on the views of the interviewee only. Different perceptions of need are catered for in separate columns, so aggregate views should not be listed in any one column. Specific differences between the scores in each of the columns (and for individual need domains) can then be used as discussion points with all relevant parties involved in the care of the individual.

Descriptions of the scoring system for each of the CANFOR scales are provided in Chapters 5–7. Not all of the need domains will be relevant to every person and/or every service environment. If particular domains are not relevant to an individual, they should be scored as 'no problem' or 'not applicable', according to the scoring criteria available for individual need domains.

4.1 Description of the Individual Need Domains

Accommodation

This domain refers to the person's current housing situation and how appropriate it is. The domain can be scored as 'not applicable' if the person is an inpatient or is in prison and is likely to remain so for the next 6 to 12 months. Alternative placement, both in the community and inpatient services, should be considered here. Unreasonable delays in securing an appropriate accommodation placement should also be considered and recorded here. What constitutes an unreasonable delay should be determined and operationalised locally.

Food

This domain refers to the person's ability to buy appropriate food and the skills to cook it by themselves. If the person is an inpatient or is in prison, this option may not be available, in which case it should be scored according to the appropriateness of the food provided by the services (either a met or an unmet need).

Looking after the Living Environment

This domain refers to the person's ability to keep their accommodation (or living space if the person is an inpatient or in prison) in a reasonable state of cleanliness. This should not necessarily be to the standard you might expect in your own home, but instead refers to basic cleanliness and tidiness.

Self-Care

This domain refers to the person's ability to keep themselves clean and tidy, in terms of bodily cleanliness and tidiness. It would therefore cover areas such as washing clothes, taking baths/showers, and shaving at regular intervals. Similar to the previous domain, ratings should reflect basic levels of personal hygiene.

Daytime Activities

This domain refers to the structure of the person's day. Daytime activities include a broad range of possible activities, including the need for, and provision of, a structured activity programme for inpatients, such as therapies, exercise and occupational therapy, further education, day-centre activities, and employment activities. Note that problems primarily due to loneliness should not be rated here, as these issues would be covered in the company domain.

Physical Health

This need domain refers to the general physical health of the person. Areas for consideration would include

routine medications/treatment required for health-related conditions, physiotherapy, operations, and side effects from any medications taken. Other areas of consideration here include problems with sleep, eyesight, hearing, and seizures.

Psychotic Symptoms

This need domain refers to any psychotic phenomena experienced by the person. Areas for consideration would include the effectiveness of psychotropic medications taken for symptomatic relief and psychological interventions provided on a one-to-one or group basis. When the person is interviewed, it is important to enquire about any medications they may be taking (if not mentioned in the previous need domain concerning physical health) and what these medications are for. If the person reports no difficulties in this domain and does not report that any medications taken are for psychotic disorders, this need domain should be scored as N (no problem).

Information about Condition and Treatment

This need domain refers to the quality, comprehensiveness, and utility of information received by the person regarding their mental health condition and any treatments that have been recommended. This information could have been received verbally or in writing. Discussion about this need domain should consider the perceived effectiveness of this information. Emphasizing that the questioning refers to difficulties and help received (and needed) in the last month is important because information might have been received in the past and the person might therefore not currently need any help in this area (in which case the need domain should be scored as no problem).

Psychological Distress

This domain refers to any 'out of the ordinary' psychological distress that may be experienced by the person. This could include adjustment difficulties, desperation, or a pervasive sense of sadness.

Safety to Self

This domain refers to self-harming behaviour and suicide attempts or intent. The need rating for this domain should be based on self-harm or suicide attempts in the last month and should include both behaviour and thinking, with consideration of the effectiveness of any interventions the person has received. The need rating for this domain should not be considered a sufficient risk assessment for care planning, so identified problems in this domain should lead to further assessment, possibly using a suitable risk assessment measure. If the person has actually self-harmed in the last month, this domain should automatically be scored as an unmet need, regardless of any subsequent preventative or therapeutic interventions.

Safety to Others

This domain refers to violent and threatening behaviour exhibited by the person towards others. The need rating should be based on any incidents that have occurred during the last month only. Completion of this need domain should not be considered a sufficient risk assessment for future violence, and any problems identified should be the basis of further investigation with an appropriate violence risk assessment measure. If the person has been violent in the last month, this domain is automatically scored as an unmet need, regardless of subsequent preventative or therapeutic interventions.

Alcohol

This domain refers to problematic alcohol use. The lack of access to alcohol, if the person is an inpatient or prisoner, might not detract from an underlying problem or need in this area.

Drugs

This domain refers to problematic drug use. The lack of access to drugs, if the person is an inpatient or prisoner, might not detract from an underlying problem or need in this area. This domain should also include consideration of the use of non-prescribed medication and the misuse of prescribed medications.

Company

This domain refers to social contacts and the ability to initiate conversation and form friendships with other people. Some people may be quite happy in their own company and may not want to socialise with others, in which case the domain should be scored as no problem.

Intimate Relationships

This domain refers to close relationships, such as with a husband, wife, or significant partner. Sensitivity may be required when exploring this and the next two need domains.

Sexual Expression

This domain refers to difficulties the person may be having with their sex lives and sexual functioning. This would include problems relating to a lack of a sex life, access to conjugal rights, and impotence (possibly due to medication side effects). Note here that if the person does not have partner, they may still have views on whether their sex life is, on balance, satisfactory or not.

Dependents (Previously Referred to as Child Care)

This domain refers to difficulties the person may be having with child care issues and/or looking after dependents. This can be particularly relevant if the person is an inpatient and family or social services are involved. This can be perceived as a sensitive domain for some people to discuss, so care should be taken when introducing the discussion topic. This domain should be scored as not applicable if the person has never had children and has no other dependents.

Basic Education

This domain refers to basic education only, such as the ability to read a shop name, complete a simple form, or count change received after purchasing something at a shop with cash. More advanced educational needs can be considered under the 'daytime activities' domain instead.

Digital Communication (Previously Telephone)

This domain refers to difficulties the person may have with being able to use a telephone or the Internet and having appropriate access to a telephone and/or online services when required. This domain can be problematic in instances where the person is in a secure psychiatric facility or prison setting where telephone and internet access are likely to be restricted or otherwise controlled.

Transport

This domain refers to difficulties the person might have with accessing transport facilities or practical difficulties associated with the use of public transport, such as reading timetables. This domain can be scored as not applicable when any difficulties have not been tested out because it is unlikely that the person in question will be using public transport in the next 6 to 12 months (the same timescale as the accommodation domain).

Money

This domain assesses budgeting skills – the basic skills required to manage money for bills, food, and so forth. If cash is not used in the service setting (e.g. in prison or secure psychiatric facility), then assessment should be based on the use of relevant acquisition forms and the extent to which budgetary considerations and limits are adhered to.

Benefits

This domain refers to difficulties the person may have with receiving the appropriate amount of benefits, according to their personal situation. Where 'traditional' benefit entitlements are not available, this domain should be scored with reference to any allowances received from services.

Treatment

This domain refers to the extent to which any treatments that are required are agreed and complied with by the person. Treatments may include medication and/or psychological interventions and supports. Consideration about whether consent to treatment details have been provided by the person can also be taken into account here.

Sexual Offences

This domain refers to prior or current problems associated with committing acts of a sexual nature. This would include inappropriate sexual behaviour, the need for sex offender treatment programmes, and so forth. This domain can be scored as not applicable if the person has no history of problems in this area and is not considered to be at current risk of committing such offences. If the person has a history of problems in this area but is not considered a current risk, then this domain should be scored as no problem. It should be noted that answers to this domain alone are not sufficient to inform risk management decisions, and problems identified should form the basis of further investigation using appropriate standardised assessment measures.

Arson

This domain refers to prior or current problems associated with the risk of setting fires. It can be scored as not applicable if the person has no history of problems in this area and is not considered to be at current risk of committing such offences. Similar to the sexual offences domain, if the person has a history of problems in this area but is not considered a current risk, then this domain should be scored as no problem. It should be noted that answers to this domain alone are not sufficient to inform risk management decisions, and problems identified should form the basis of further investigation using appropriate risk assessment measures.

4.2 Guidance for Interviewing

The interviewer should be a professional with some knowledge of the difficulties that can be involved in interviewing someone with serious mental illness. Issues relating to personal safety and confidentiality should also be considered, and recommendations should be complied with.

When assessing the person, it is recommended that the interview commences with an overview of the purpose of the assessment and a brief description of the structure of the assessment. It would be appropriate to explain the format that the assessment will take and how the questions are structured. It is also a good idea to explain that some of the areas will not be relevant for the person in question and that some of the questions cover some more personal areas that they may decide they do not wish to discuss. One such approach to introducing the assessment process for CANFOR could be as follows:

"This assessment asks a number of questions about areas that people can sometimes have difficulties with. There are 25 broad areas of need to cover, and some of them may not be relevant or applicable to you. Each question follows exactly the same format, starting by asking if you have had any difficulties in the area, then focusing on difficulties you may have experienced in the last month. If you have experienced any difficulties in this area, I would then like to ask you about any help you have been receiving, firstly from friends and family, then from health/social/welfare and other support services; what help you need from these services; and finally, how satisfied you are with the help that you have been receiving from services during the last month. We will go through each question in turn, so please let me know if there is anything you do not

understand, and as I mentioned before, if there are questions that you would prefer not to answer, please say so and we can move on to the next question."

You should also give some indication about how long the interview will take in total. Generally speaking, a full assessment (using the CANFOR-C or CANFOR-R) will take 20–25 minutes to complete, while the short version (CANFOR-S) will take up to 15 minutes to complete. Each of the need domains are self-contained, so breaks can be taken as required and a full assessment can be completed over more than one sitting if necessary.

All questions should be phrased simply and unambiguously. Each need domain provides introductory 'trigger' questions that seek to open discussions about a particular topic. It is highly likely that further questions will be required before a need rating can be decided upon and the next need domain can be considered. These further questions should seek to focus the area of discussion and to identify whether any help is currently being received and, if so, to what extent it is helping. These questions should also aim to identify what help the person might need for particular problems/difficulties and, in general, how satisfied they are with the level and type of help received in this area. It is important to reiterate that the timeframe of interest here to make a need rating for each domain focuses on problems/difficulties experienced during the past month only.

Note: The opening questioning may appear to indicate that there are no difficulties in the domain, so the interviewer may be inclined to record this as no need and move on to the next domain. However, there may be no difficulties in the domain because of the help that the person has been receiving for their difficulties in this area. Therefore, it is always necessary to differentiate between situations where the person has no problems and needs no help in the domain (no problem) from those where the person would have difficulties were it not for the help that they have been receiving (a met need).

The CANFOR domains are ordered in such a way as to leave more personal difficulties (i.e. those of a more sensitive nature) to later on in the interview, when both the interviewer and interviewee are familiar with the types and style of questioning. All 25 domains should be assessed when completing a CANFOR assessment, but the order that the domains are assessed can be flexible. For example, difficulties may be raised by the interviewee in a domain that is not routinely asked about until later in the assessment, and the interviewer may choose to move on to that domain, and then go back and assess and complete the intervening domains.

4.3 Suggested Questioning Process for Each Domain on All CANFOR Scales

1. Historically, has there been a problem in this particular area?

2. Has this been the case during the last month?

3. Does the person need any help for this problem at the moment?

4. Are they receiving any help (informal or formal) at the moment?

5. Is any help that they are receiving actually helping and, if so, how much?

6. (*For service-user interviews*) Is the interviewee satisfied with the help they are receiving at the moment for this particular problem? (*Then, for staff interviews, where indicated*) Did problems in this area contribute to the index offence or reasons for referral to the service?

The first question seeks to introduce the interviewee to the general domain area. The second question then focuses the discussions on problems/difficulties experienced during the last month (i.e. the time frame of interest). The third and fourth questions seek to determine the extent of any current problems experienced and to enquire about any help that is currently being received for these difficulties. The fifth question then seeks to determine the perceived effectiveness of the current help being received and should then go on to enquire about possible discrepancies between what the person is currently receiving and what help is currently needed. The sixth question seeks to summarise discussions and should inform the overall need rating for each domain.

Once these six questions have been covered, it should be possible to make an informed need rating for the domain area. Each domain is structured in the same way and is self-contained, allowing for breaks to be taken during the interview if and when necessary.

Using the Camberwell Assessment of Need Forensic Research Version (CANFOR-R)

The CANFOR-R is a semi-structured interview schedule, assessing need in 25 domains of the person's life, suitable for research purposes. Need domains cover a range of psychological, social, clinical, and functional needs, reflecting the broad range of needs a person can have. Each domain is structured the same and is self-contained, thereby allowing for breaks to be taken during the interview if necessary. Each domain has four sections, which are described below. The CANFOR-R is meant for research purposes and covers needs/problems *in the past month only*. A full clinical version (CANFOR-C) and a short one-page summary version (CANFOR-S) are also available. Brief details of how to complete the assessment, along with a copy of the scale, are included in Appendix 1.

5.1 Section 1

This section is meant to introduce the domain to the interviewee and is used to open discussion on that topic. It aims to summarise the presence or absence of a need in the particular domain and, if present, whether the perceived need is met or unmet by current supports and interventions. Before deciding on a need rating for the section, it is usually necessary to consider the questions raised in the other sections of the page. This is especially the case where the interviewee reports that there are no problems/difficulties in the area, but this actually may be because they are receiving appropriate 'helpful' help for the difficulties they have in the domain. If you do not go on to ask about any help being received in the area over the last month, which may account for why the person reports there currently being no problem, an inaccurate need score would be made. Five possible scoring options are available for Section 1, as follows:

5.1.1 Rating a Domain as No Need (Indicated by 'N')

A rating of no problem would indicate that the person does not currently have any problems/difficulties in the domain and that they are not currently receiving any help in this area. An example could be where someone reports that they have not been violent in the last month and have not been receiving any interventions or supports (preventative or therapeutic) in this area. Additionally, no need would be scored where a person reports that they do not have any problems with alcohol consumption and that they have not been receiving any help, supports, or interventions for problems/difficulties in the area.

5.1.2 Rating a Domain as a Met Need (Indicated by 'M')

A rating of a met need would indicate that the person currently has some problems/difficulties in the domain and that effective help is being received. For example, a met need could be indicated where the person reports difficulties with psychotic symptoms, that they are receiving medication and/or other therapeutic/supportive help for those difficulties, and that this help is effective. Similarly, a met need would be indicated where the person reports difficulties with daytime activities and that they have been attending a day centre, education classes, or other therapeutic/supportive activities that have effectively reduced the difficulties they have been experiencing in this area.

5.1.3 Rating a Domain as an Unmet Need (Indicated by 'U')

A rating of an unmet need would indicate that the person currently has some difficulties/problems in the domain and either that they are not getting any help at all for these problems, or that any help being received is not effective. For example, an unmet need is indicated in a situation where the person reports difficulties/problems with psychological distress and doesn't perceive that any of the interventions/supports they have been receiving have been effective (i.e. that the help is not helping, and their difficulties remain significant). Similarly, an unmet need would be indicated where the person reports that they have some difficulties with their physical health and that they are not receiving any treatments/supports that help, so the domain remains a significant ongoing problem for them.

5.1.4 Rating a Domain as Not Applicable (Indicated by 'NA')

A rating of not applicable is only available for five of the CANFOR-R domains. For the sexual offending and arson domains, a not applicable score can be made if the person has no history of problems/difficulties in the area and reports no current problems/difficulties in the area. The accommodation domain can be scored as not applicable if the person is currently an inpatient/prisoner who is not likely to be transferred/discharged/released in the next 6 to 12 months. Transport can be scored as not applicable according to the same criteria as the accommodation domain. Dependents can be scored as not applicable if the person has never had children (including adopted children) and has no other dependents. None of the other CANFOR-R domains should be scored as not applicable.

5.1.5 Rating a Domain as Not Known (Indicated by '?')

A rating of not known can be scored when the person being interviewed either does not know (or is not confident in their answer) or does not wish to disclose any information about any problems/difficulties they might be aware of. An example of scoring a domain as not known could be where the interviewee did not wish to answer questions about any problems/difficulties they may be having in the sexual expression domain, as they perhaps felt it was a personal matter. Alternatively, in the case of an interview with a staff member or carer, a score of not known could be recorded if they were not entirely sure if the person was having current problems/difficulties in the area, as they had perhaps not discussed this area with them.

5.2 Section 2

This section assesses the level of help that is being received from informal sources. Informal sources include family, friends, and neighbours. This help can cover a broad range of supportive help, as well as more specific hands-on interventions. For example, regular telephone calls from family or friends may be perceived as effective help for certain problems/difficulties such as psychological distress. It can be beneficial for the interviewer to personalise the questions if the interviewee mentions particular names of friends or family members, but be careful to not limit discussions to these named persons, as other informal types of help may be being received as well. It may well be the case that different people help with different types of problems/difficulties, so it is important to try to capture the full range of supports the person may be receiving. Note here that we do not ask how much help is needed from these informal sources, as this could be perceived critically. Section 2 of the CANFOR-R is scored according to a sliding scale.

0 = no help	Indicates that no help was received from informal sources for this domain.
1 = low help	Indicates that the interviewee thought that any help received was only helping a small amount. An example commonly used for this would be where brief advice or leaflets were given to the person concerning any difficulties the person had in the domain.
2 = medium help	Indicates that the interview thought that any help being received was helping moderately. An example commonly used here could be more regular structured support, at least on a weekly basis.
3 = high help	Indicates that the interviewee thought that the help being received was helping substantially. An example of this could be the provision of a structured intervention/support, or daily input and/or supervision.
? = not known / prefer not to say	Indicates that the interviewee did not know to what degree any interventions/supports were helping with the particular problems/difficulties in the domain, or perhaps that they did not want to disclose any information on this topic.

It should be noted here that these scores and exemplars are only meant as indicators and suggested anchor points; it is likely that responses will not directly refer to the examples provided here. A value judgment is therefore necessary when scoring this section of CANFOR-R. It is also important to remember that even if highly intensive support/interventions have been provided, the interviewee may not feel that they are helping at all (or to the degree that perhaps they should). In these circumstances, the rating should reflect the degree to which the interviewee perceives the help to be helping. Note that the interviewee is not asked whether they need anything in addition, or as an alternative, to any informal help being received.

5.3 Section 3

Section 3 has two purposes in that it is used to determine the current and required levels of help needed from services. Firstly, it considers the level of help received from services over the last month. Then, secondly, it assesses that person's need for help in the domain. The two questions utilise the same rating scale based upon the suggested anchor points. Section 3 of the CANFOR-R is scored according to a sliding scale:

0 = no help	Indicates that the interviewee thought that no help was received from services.
1 = low help	Indicates that the interviewee thought that any help received from services was only helping a small amount.
2 = medium help	Indicates that the interviewee thought that any help being received from services was helping moderately.
3 = high help	Indicates that the interviewee thought that the help being received from services was helping substantially.
? = not known/ prefer not to say	Indicates that the interviewee did not know to what degree any interventions/supports being received from services were helping with the particular problems/ difficulties in the domain, or perhaps that they did not want to disclose any information on this topic.

Again, it should be noted here that these scores and examples are only meant as anchor points and responses will commonly not directly refer to the example provided. As such, a certain value judgment is necessary when scoring this section of the CANFOR-R. The rating recorded here should directly reflect the degree to which the interviewee perceives the help received to be helping them (or the

person the staff member or family member is being interviewed about); this is not necessarily reflective of the frequency or intensity of the interventions themselves.

The second part of Section 3 considers what help is actually needed from services for each of the need domains. An important point to emphasize during the interview is that this focuses on what is needed as opposed to what is wanted; these two concepts can be quite different. This rating is made using the same sliding scale with reference to the anchor points, ranging from no help through to high help. In terms of interpretation, if the same rating is recorded in Section 3 for help received and help needed, this would suggest that appropriate levels and types of help were being received. However, if the score is higher for help needed over help being received, this may indicate an unmet need in the domain. It may also be the case that the interviewee reports that a different type of help is needed and that the current interventions received from services are ineffective; in this case, the current help received would likely be scored as 0 (no help) and the help needed as 3 (high help).

5.4 Section 4

This final section of each CANFOR-R domain also has two purposes. Firstly, it considers how satisfied overall the person is with any help that has been received from services over the last month. This question is asked of the service user only and can be scored as:

NS = not satisfied	Overall, the person is not satisfied with the help that they have received from services over the last month.
S = satisfied	Overall, the person is satisfied with the help that has been received from services over the last month.
? = not known/ prefer not to say	The person does not know or does not want to answer this question.

Secondly, for 16 of the 25 need domains, the staff member is asked whether any problems/difficulties experienced by the person in these domains may have contributed to their index offence or reasons leading to referral/transfer to the service. This question serves an important purpose. If it is recorded that problems/difficulties in the area contributed at all to any of the 16 domains considered, further assessment and consideration should be given to better understand the gravity and nature of these issues. It could indicate, for example, that the need domain is an area for priority action in terms of care planning, treatment, and/or specialist assessment. Possible scoring options for this last section of the CANFOR-R are:

0 = not at all	Problems/difficulties in the area did not contribute at all to the index offence or reasons for referral to the service.
1 = a little bit	Problems/difficulties in the area contributed a small amount to the index offence or reasons for referral to the service.
2 = substantially	Problems/difficulties in the area contributed significantly to the index offence or reasons for referral to the service.
? = not known/ prefer not to say	The person does not know, is not sure, or does not want to answer whether problems/difficulties they experienced in the area contributed to their index offence or reasons for referral to the service.

Note: In addition, for the accommodation domain, the staff member is also asked if there have been unreasonable delays in transferring the person to more appropriate accommodation (prison transfer, hospital transfer, or community placement). While this should be determined locally, the general principle applied has been that a wait of more than one month constitutes an unreasonable delay. Also, note that the lack of availability of an appropriate placement is not considered when recording responses to this question.

5.5 Using Information from a CANFOR-R Assessment

CANFOR-R can be used as an outcome measure for research purposes at both individual and service levels. One such use could be investigating the extent to which informal and formal sources of help continue to meet the needs of the person in different service environments.

Using the Camberwell Assessment of Need Forensic Clinical Version (CANFOR-C)

CANFOR-C is a semi-structured interview schedule, assessing need in 25 domains of the person's life, suitable for clinical use. Need domains cover a range of psychological, social, clinical, and functional needs, reflecting the broad range of needs a person can have. Each domain is structured the same and is self-contained, thereby allowing for breaks to be taken during the interview if necessary. Each domain has four sections, which are described below. CANFOR-C is meant for clinical use and covers needs/problems *in the past month only*. A full research version (CANFOR-R) and a short one-page summary version (CANFOR-S) are also available. Brief details of how to complete the assessment, along with a copy of the scale, are included in Appendix 2.

6.1 Section 1

This section is meant to introduce the domain to the interviewee and is used to open discussion on that topic. It aims to summarise the presence or absence of a need in the particular domain and, if present, whether the perceived need is met or unmet by current supports and interventions. Before deciding on a need rating for the section, it is usually necessary to consider the questions raised in the other sections of the page. This is especially the case where the interviewee reports that there are no problems/difficulties in the area, but this is actually because they are receiving appropriate help for the difficulties they have in the domain. If you do not go on to ask about any help being received over the last month, which may account for why the person reports there currently being no problem, an inaccurate need score would be made. Five possible scoring options are available for Section 1:

6.1.1 Rating a Domain as No Need (Indicated by 'N')

A rating of no problem would indicate that the person does not currently have any problems/difficulties in

the domain and that they are not currently receiving any help in this area. An example could be where someone reports that they have not been violent in the last month and have not been receiving any interventions or supports (preventative or therapeutic) in this area. Additionally, a rating of no need would be indicated where a person reports that they do not have any problems with alcohol consumption and that they have not been receiving any help, supports, or interventions for problems/difficulties in the area.

6.1.2 Rating a Domain as a Met Need (Indicated by 'M')

A rating of a met need would indicate that the person currently has some problems/difficulties in the domain and that effective help is being received. For example, a met need could be indicated where the person reports difficulties with psychotic symptoms, that they are receiving medication and/or other therapeutic/supportive help for those difficulties, and that this help is effective for them. Similarly, a met need would be indicated where the person reports difficulties with daytime activities and that they have been attending a day centre, education classes, or other therapeutic/supportive activities that have effectively reduced the difficulties they have been experiencing in this area.

6.1.3 Rating a Domain as an Unmet Need (Indicated by 'U')

A rating of an unmet need would indicate that the person currently has some difficulties/problems in the domain and either that they are not getting any help at all for these problems or that any help being received is not effective. For example, an unmet need is indicated in a situation where the person reports difficulties/problems with psychological distress and doesn't perceive that any of the interventions/supports they have been receiving have been effective (i.e. that the help is not helping and the difficulties remain significant). Similarly, an unmet need would be indicated where the person reports that they have some difficulties with their physical health and that they are not receiving any treatments/supports that help, so the domain remains a significant ongoing problem for them.

6.1.4 Rating a Domain as Not Applicable (Indicated by 'NA')

A rating of not applicable is only available for five of the CANFOR-C domains. For the sexual offending and arson domains, a not applicable score can be made if the person has no history of problems/difficulties in the area and reports no current problems/difficulties in the respective areas. The accommodation domain can be scored as not applicable if the person is currently an inpatient/prisoner who is not likely to be transferred/discharged/released in the next 6 to 12 months. Transport is scored as not applicable according to the same criteria as the accommodation domain. Dependents can be scored as not applicable if the person has never had children (including adopted children) and has no other dependents. None of the other CANFOR-C domains should be scored as not applicable.

6.1.5 Rating a Domain as Not Known (Indicated by '?')

A rating of not known can be scored when the person being interviewed either does not know (or is not confident in their answer) or does not wish to disclose any information about any problems/difficulties they might be aware of. An example of scoring a domain as not known could be where the interviewee did not wish to answer questions about any problems/difficulties they may be having in the sexual expression domain, as they perhaps felt it was a personal matter. Alternatively, in the case of an interview with a staff member or carer, a score of not known could be recorded if they were not entirely sure if the person was having current problems/difficulties in the area, as they have perhaps not discussed this area with them.

6.2 Section 2

This section assesses the level of help that is being received from informal sources. Informal sources include family, friends, and neighbours. This help can cover a broad range of supportive help, as well as more specific hands-on interventions. For example, regular telephone calls from family or friends may be perceived as effective help for certain problems/difficulties such as psychological distress. It can be beneficial for the interviewer to personalise the questions if the interviewee mentions particular names of friends or family members, but be careful to not limit discussions to these named persons, as other informal help may be being received as well. It may well be the case that different people help with different types of problems/difficulties, so it is important to try to capture the full range of supports the person may be receiving. Note here that we do not ask how much help is needed from these informal sources, as this could be perceived critically. Section 2 of the CANFOR-C is scored according to a sliding scale.

0 = no help	Indicates that no help was received from informal sources for this domain.
1 = low help	Indicates that the interviewee thought that any help received was only helping a small amount. An example commonly used for this would be where brief advice or leaflets were given to the person concerning any difficulties the person had in the domain.
2 = medium help	Indicates that the interview thought that any help being received was helping moderately. An example commonly used here could be more regular structured support, at least on a weekly basis.
3 = high help	Indicates that the interviewee thought that the help being received was helping substantially. An example of this could be the provision of a structured intervention/support, or daily input and/or supervision.
? = not known/ prefer not to say	Indicates that the interviewee did not know to what degree any interventions/supports were helping with the particular problems/difficulties in the domain, or perhaps that they did not want to disclose any information on this topic.

It should be noted here that these scores and exemplars are only meant as indicators and suggested anchor points; it is likely that responses will not directly refer to the examples provided here. A value judgment is therefore necessary when scoring this section of CANFOR-C. It is also important to remember that even if a highly intensive support/intervention has been provided, the interviewee may not feel that it is helping at all (or to the degree that perhaps it should). In these circumstances, the rating should reflect the degree to which the interviewee perceives the help to be helping. Note that the interviewee is not asked whether they need anything in addition, or as an alternative, to any informal help being received.

6.3 Section 3

Section 3 has two purposes in that it is used to determine the current and required levels of help needed from services. Firstly, it considers the level of help received from services over the last month. Then, secondly, it assesses that person's need for help in the domain. The two questions utilise the same rating scale based upon the suggested anchor points. Section 3 of the CANFOR-C is scored according to a sliding scale:

0 = no help	Indicates that the interviewee thought that no help was received from services.
1 = low help	Indicates that the interviewee thought that any help received from services was only helping a small amount.
2 = medium help	Indicates that the interviewee thought that any help being received from services was helping moderately.
3 = high help	Indicates that the interviewee thought that the help being received from services was helping substantially.
? = not known / prefer not to say	Indicates that the interviewee did not know to what degree any interventions/supports being received from services were helping with the particular problems/difficulties in the domain, or perhaps that they did not want to disclose any information on this topic.

Again, it should be noted here that these scores and examples are only meant as anchor points and responses will commonly not directly refer to the example provided. As such, a certain value judgment is necessary when scoring this section of the CANFOR-C. The rating recorded here should directly reflect the degree to which the interviewee perceives help being received to be helping them (or the person the staff member or family member is being interviewed about); this is not necessarily reflective of the frequency or intensity of the interventions themselves.

The second part of Section 3 considers what help is actually needed from services for each of the need domains. An important point to emphasize during the interview is that this focuses on what is needed as opposed to what is wanted; these two concepts can be quite different. This rating is made using the same sliding scale with reference to the anchor points ranging from 'no help' through to 'high help'. In terms of interpretation, if the same rating is recorded in Section 3 for help received and help needed, this would suggest that appropriate levels and types of help were being received. However, if the score is higher for help needed over help being received, this could indicate an unmet need in the domain. It may also be the case that the interviewee reports that a different type of help is needed and that the current interventions received from services are ineffective; in this case, the current help received would likely be scored as 0 (no help) and the help needed as a 3 (high help).

6.4 Section 4

This final section of each CANFOR-C domain also has two purposes. Firstly, it considers how satisfied overall the person is with any help that has been received from services over the last month. This question is asked of the service user only and can be scored as:

NS = not satisfied	Overall, the person is not satisfied with the help that they have received from services over the last month.
S = satisfied	Overall, the person is satisfied with the help that has been received from services over the last month.
? = not known/ prefer not to say	The person does not know or does not want to answer this question.

Secondly, at the bottom of the page, there are boxes providing space for notes regarding possible interventions for difficulties identified in each need domain and appropriate action points and review dates. Consideration should be given, where appropriate, to whether problems/difficulties in the individual need domains may have contributed to the index offence/reason for referral to the service. In addition, notes relating to risks, proximity to family, restrictions, relapse indicators, and discrepancies between viewpoints should be recorded here and form the basis of extended discussions. In addition, for the accommodation domain, any unreasonable delays in transferring the person to a more appropriate accommodation (whether a community, hospital, or prison placement) should be recorded. The general principle applied here is that a wait exceeding one month constitutes an unreasonable delay.

6.5 Using Information from a CANFOR-C Assessment

CANFOR-C can be used at both individual and service levels. On an individual level, CANFOR-C can be used as an in-depth baseline indicator of need when entering a service and then subsequently to monitor change and progress over time, as well as helping to gauge the perceived effectiveness of supports and interventions the person receives. At a service level, CANFOR-C data can be used for auditing and developing specific services. For example, aggregate measures of need in key domains may inform the need for additional services or multi-agency collaborations, or to measure the impact of service-based group interventions.

Using the Camberwell Assessment of Need Forensic Short Version (CANFOR-S)

CANFOR-S is a semi-structured interview schedule, assessing need in 25 domains of the person's life. Unlike CANFOR-R and CANFOR-C, this version is a short, one-page summary of the need domains. It summarises the need score for each domain area, along with whether problems/difficulties in each of the domains contributed to the index offence/reasons for referral to the service. Brief details of how to complete the assessment, along with a copy of the scale, are included in Appendix 3.

The presence or absence of a need is identified for each of the 25 need domains and, if present, whether the perceived need is met or unmet by current interventions. Before deciding on a need rating, it is recommended that the interviewer considers the question areas raised in each of the other sections of the full CANFOR-R or CANFOR-C (i.e. sections 2, 3, and 4). It is therefore recommended that interviewers are familiar with the content and questioning style of the CANFOR-R and CANFOR-C and keep a copy of one of the full versions with them for reference when interviewing and completing the CANFOR-S.

A shorter questioning process is feasible for CANFOR-S, as follows:

1. During the last month, have you had any problems in this area?
2. If no, is this because of any help you are currently receiving for these problems?
3. On balance, would you say that this is still a serious problem for you?
4. (*For staff interviews only*) Do you think that problems in this area contributed to the index offence/reasons for referral to the service?

Suggesting opening trigger questions are provided in italics for each need domain; these need to be adjusted slightly and rephrased, depending on who you are interviewing, to personalise the interview to their perception (e.g. staff and carer perspectives). Note here that it is likely that further questions will be necessary to focus the discussion on

difficulties experienced specifically in the last month. Consider what help has been received, what help is needed, and (for service users) their overall satisfaction with help received. Five possible scoring options are available for the need rating for each domain.

7.1 Rating a Domain as No Need (Indicated by 'N')

A rating of no need would indicate that the person does not currently have any problems/difficulties in the domain and that they are not currently receiving any help in this area. An example could be where someone reports that they have not been violent in the last month and have not been receiving any interventions or supports (preventative or therapeutic) in this area. Additionally, no need would be scored where a person reports that they do not have any problems with alcohol consumption and that they have not been receiving any help, supports or interventions for problems/difficulties in the area.

7.2 Rating a Domain as a Met Need (Indicated by 'M')

A rating of a met need would indicate that the person currently has some problems/difficulties in the domain and that effective help is being received. For example, a met need could be indicated where the person reports difficulties with psychotic symptoms, that they are receiving medication and/or other therapeutic/supportive help for those difficulties, and that this help is effective for them. Similarly, a met need would be indicated where the person reports difficulties with daytime activities and that they have been attending a day centre, education classes, or other therapeutic/supportive activities that have effectively reduced the difficulties they have been experiencing in this area.

7.3 Rating a Domain as an Unmet Need (Indicated by 'U')

A rating of an unmet need would indicate that the person currently has some difficulties/problems in the domain and either that they are not getting any help at all for these problems or that any help being received is not effective. For example, an unmet need is indicated in a situation where the person reports difficulties/problems with psychological distress and doesn't perceive that any of the interventions/supports they have been receiving have been effective (i.e. that the help is not helping and the difficulties remain significant). Similarly, an unmet need would be indicated where the person reports that they have some difficulties with their physical health and that they are not receiving any treatments/supports that help, so the domain remains a significant ongoing problem for them.

7.4 Rating a Domain as Not Applicable (Indicated by 'NA')

A rating of not applicable is only available for five of the CANFOR-S domains. For the sexual offending and arson domains, a not applicable score can be made if the person has no history of problems/difficulties in the area and reports no current problems/difficulties in the respective areas. The accommodation domain can be scored as not applicable if the person is currently an inpatient/prisoner who is not likely to be transferred/discharged/released in the next 6 to 12 months. Transport is scored as not applicable according to the same criteria as the accommodation domain. Dependents can be scored as not applicable if the person has never had children (including adopted children) and has no other dependents. None of the other CANFOR-S domains should be scored as not applicable.

7.5 Rating a Domain as Not Known (Indicated by '?')

A rating of not known can be scored when the person being interviewed either does not know (or is not confident in their answer) or does not wish to disclose any information about any problems/difficulties they might be aware of. An example of scoring a domain as not known could be where the interviewee did not wish to answer questions about any problems/difficulties they may be having in the sexual expression domain, as they perhaps felt it was a personal matter. Alternatively, in the case of an interview with a staff member or carer, a score of not known could be recorded if they were not entirely sure if the person was having current problems/difficulties in the area, as they may have not discussed this area with them (or at least done so recently – in the last month).

Secondly, for 16 of the 25 need domains, the staff member is asked whether any problems/difficulties experienced by the person in these domains may have contributed to their index offence or reasons leading to referral/transfer to the service (far right column of CANFOR-S). This question serves an important purpose. If it is recorded that problems/difficulties in the area contributed at all to any of the 16 domains considered, further assessment and consideration should be given to better understand the gravity and nature of these issues. It could indicate, for example, that the need domain is an area for priority action in terms of care planning, treatment, and/or specialist assessment. Possible scoring options for this last column on the CANFOR-S are:

Yes	Problems/difficulties in the area did contribute to the index offence or reasons for referral to the service.
No	Problems/difficulties in the area did not contribute to the index offence or reasons for referral to the service.
?	The person does not know, is not sure, or does not want to answer whether problems/difficulties they experienced in the area contributed to their index offence or reasons for referral to the service.

Translations of the CANFOR

The CANFOR has successfully been translated into several other languages, including Spanish, Italian, Portuguese, Japanese, French, and Swedish. For further details, or if you are interested in translating the CANFOR into other languages, please contact Professor Stuart Thomas in the first instance.

To date, three of these collaborations have led to peer-reviewed outputs being published: a Spanish version, a Portuguese version, and an Italian version. Brief details about these projects are provided as follows.

8.1 Spanish Version of the CANFOR

The CANFOR has been translated into Spanish, with a paper describing its psychometric properties being published in 2010. The study was based upon administering the CANFOR to 90 service users who had been diagnosed with a severe mental disorder and had been admitted to prison. Further details can be found in the following publication, as follows:

Romeva, G.E., Rubio, L.G., Guerre, S.O., Miravet, M. J., Caceres, A.G., & Thomas, S.D. (2010). Clinical validation of the CANFOR scale (Camberwell Assessment of Need Forensic Version) for the needs assessment of people with mental health problems in the forensic services, *Actas, Esp Psiquiatr, 38*, 129–137.

8.2 Portuguese Version of the CANFOR

The CANFOR has been translated into Portuguese, with a paper describing its psychometric properties being published in 2013. The study was based on interviews with 143 service users and their case managers across four different forensic mental health services in and around the city of Lisbon. Further details can be found in the publication, as follows:

Talina, M., Thomas, S., Cardoso, A., Aguiar, P., Caldas de Almeida, J.M., & Xavier, M. (2013). CANFOR Portuguese version: validation study. *BMC Psychiatry, 13*, 157. DOI: 10.1186/1471-244X-13-157

8.3 Italian Version of the CANFOR

The CANFOR has been translated into Italian, with a paper describing its psychometric properties being published in 2014. The study was based on staff ratings of 50 forensic mental health service users from a high-security psychiatric hospital in Northern Italy. Further details can be found in the publication, as follows:

Castelletti, L., Lasavlia, A., Molinari, E., & Thomas, S.D. M., Stratico, E., & Bonetto, C. (2014). A standardised tool for assessing needs in forensic psychiatric populations: clinical validation of the Italian CANFOR, staff version. *Epidemiology and Psychiatric Services, 24*, 274–281. DOI: 10.1017/S2045796014000602

Suggested Training

What follows are guidance notes for a training session in the use of the CANFOR scales for clinical staff and researchers. A brief structural plan for the session is outlined, as well as some suggested summary points that could be converted into slides/handouts. These can also readily be adapted to the local environment and conditions.

The following points can be used as the basis for a training session to help familiarise people with the concept of needs assessment and to provide some practical experience with completing a CANFOR assessment. Although extensive formal training is generally not necessary, an initial session such as this can be used to discuss why the CANFOR assessments are being introduced, what their purpose will be, and what will be expected of people who will be completing the assessments. Training sessions will also serve to increase the consistency and reliability of the CANFOR assessments that are completed.

The training session should be informal and as interactive as possible. It should be facilitated by someone with sufficient practical experience of completing the CANFOR assessments in the setting where the staff/researchers will be working. In terms of resourcing a training session, trainers should have a sufficient number of copies of each of the CANFOR scales, summary score sheets and practice vignettes, and a means of noting key discussion points (e.g. flip chart with stand, post-it notes).

The materials provided here equate to a half-day training. Time should be made available for active discussion by participants as this will help consolidate their learning and become more confident with completing the CANFOR assessments by themselves. A brief follow-up review session should be factored in with group participants to help identify any practical challenges in completing the CANFOR assessments in practice and to help iron out any errors in scoring or interpretation that may creep in as they start to use the assessments.

9.1 Aims of Session

- What is a need?
- Why assess need?
- How do we assess need?
- Practicalities and using the CANFOR assessments

Issues to Consider (Suggested Time, 15 Minutes)

It is recommended that the session starts with introducing the concept of need itself, reasons why we need to assess needs, and generating some ideas about different ways needs can be assessed. Details provided in the earlier chapters of the book could be used by way of introduction here. It is also important to discuss the reasons that the CANFOR assessments are being used and introduced into the service or the research project.

9.2 Initial Considerations

- List as many different needs as you can.
- What are some differences between a need and an intervention?
- What needs are considered universal? What additional needs and wider considerations are potentially relevant for forensic mental health service users?

Issues to Consider (Suggested Time, 15 Minutes)

It can be useful to ask the staff (or researchers) to think of as many needs as they can so as to generate a broad list of areas that could be considered in a needs assessment. It is then important to get people to think about potential differences between a need and an intervention. For example, a person does not have a need for psychological therapy, as this is only one of a number of possible interventions for a particular problem. It is also recommended to discuss wider considerations of needs assessments in forensic services, such as security needs, political profile, and risk.

9.3 The Concept of Need in Mental Health

- The majority of people who experience severe mental illness may well have multiple or complex needs requiring access to, and support from, a number of services at any one time.
- It is highly likely that a multi-agency response will be required to fully meet their needs.
- Needs change over time, depending on different situations and circumstances.
- It is vital to be able to identify all needs at any given time, so that the most appropriate types and levels of help can be provided.
- Incorporate the personal choice of the person with professional views, in the context of wider public safety and risk management issues.
- Consider need as a subjective concept (i.e. that different people may well have different, and yet equally valid, views about the presence or absence of a need).

Issues to Consider (Suggested Time, 10 Minutes)

We must be able to measure, or otherwise account for, changing patterns of need in terms of monitoring progress and measuring service needs, as well as monitoring the need to refer people for specific interventions provided by other services (such as psychology, welfare benefits, or drug/alcohol issues).

Need is a subjective concept; people may well have different views about the presence of a need, but all of these views should be considered as being valid and should be considered when completing a comprehensive assessment. These different viewpoints are accommodated in the CANFOR scales in separate columns; these should be recorded separately and not be combined when completing the scales. When the views from different sources have been collected, the need ratings can be used as the basis of planning care and treatment packages, and then monitored with subsequent reviews to assess progress and review the perceived effectiveness of interventions provided to the person over time.

9.4 Introducing the Full CANFOR Sections

- Section 1 acts as a filter to determine the need for further assessment. It introduces the need domain to the interviewee and ultimately *provides the overall need rating* for the domain.
- Section 2 considers how much informal help from friends and family has been received during the last month.
- Section 3 considers current and required levels of help from services. It rates perceived levels of help received and the interviewee's perception of what help they actually need.
- Section 4 has two purposes. It assesses the service user's overall satisfaction with the help they are currently receiving and, where indicated, the staff member is also asked if problems/difficulties in the area may have contributed to the index offence or reasons that the person was referred to the service.

Issues to Consider (Suggested Time, 15 Minutes)

Emphasize that all 25 CANFOR domains assess need in a systematic way and a consistent flow to questioning is provided, with the same types of questions being asked for each need domain. As such, the full scales (CANFOR-R and CANFOR-C) are not as daunting as they may initially appear. Also emphasize that when completing the short version (CANFOR-S), the same range of questions needs to be asked in order to complete an informed need rating for each domain.

As an exercise here, show participants a page from either the CANFOR-R or CANFOR-C and orientate them to the layout of the need domains. This will help familiarise participants with how to navigate the page and ask the questions in the proposed sequence, in addition to demonstrating where to find trigger questions and how to choose the most appropriate option, based on the anchor points provided, that best reflects the persons' responses. Separately show the CANFOR-S layout, pointing out the columns to be completed that provide space for staff, service user, and carer perspectives, as well as the 'Contribution to the Index Offence' column.

9.5 Pointers for Completion

- Use the full clinical version (CANFOR-C) when first assessing the person; then use the short summary version (CANFOR-S) for reviews on a regular basis, where appropriate.

- Record the interviewee's perspective directly, even if it differs from your own or from what other people have reported.
- Use the summary results to discuss treatment/ intervention and support options with the person.

Issues to Consider (Suggested Time, 15 Minutes)

The most important point to be emphasized here is that *the interviewee's viewpoint is recorded directly*. This can be harder to do than you may first think. The discrepancies between different viewpoints can be useful in terms of care/treatment planning and actively involving the person in their support, care, and treatment options.

9.6 Flow of Questioning

- Historically, **has there ever been a problem** in this particular area?
- Has this been the case **over the past month**?
- Do they **need** any help for this problem at the moment?
- Are they **receiving** any help (informal or formal) at the moment?
- Is any help that they are currently receiving from services **actually helping** and, if so,
  how much?
- (*For the service user viewpoint*) Overall, **how satisfied** are they with the help they have been receiving in this area over the last month? (*For the staff viewpoint*) Did problems/ difficulties in this area **contribute to the person's index offence or reason for referral to the service**?

Issues to Consider (Suggested Time, 5 Minutes)

There is a logical flow to questioning that is replicated in each of the need domains. Following this structure and sequence allows the rater to introduce the area to the interviewee, then focus on difficulties experienced over the last month (the time frame of interest), and then judge the perceived effectiveness of any help being received. Using this questioning style will also lead to more consistent completion of the assessment by different staff and/ or researchers.

9.7 Scoring and Interpretation (Section 1: Overall Need Rating for Domain)

N = no problem	No problems/difficulties in the area during the last month and not receiving any help in this area.
M = met need	Has problems/difficulties, receiving effective 'helpful' help.
U = unmet need	Has problems/difficulties, not receiving any help, or help received not helping.
NA = not applicable	An option for five of the CANFOR domains (see individual domains for further guidance here).
? = not known/ prefer not to say	Respondent does not know or does not want to answer.

Issues to Consider (Suggested Time, 10 Minutes)

This introduces people to the overall need rating score for each CANFOR domain. Relating these scores to a particular CANFOR domain will help familiarise them with the scales. It is important to note that the not applicable response is only available for 5 of the 25 need domains and to highlight these five domains to them. It would also be useful to emphasize here that in this 2nd edition of CANFOR, we have moved away from numeric scoring and replaced this with a simpler letter-based scoring system to denote whether there is a need and if it is met or unmet. We have found that this revised recording of the overall need rating provides a much more readily accessible summary to interpret in routine use.

9.8 Scoring and Interpretation (Sections 2 and 3 of CANFOR-R and CANFOR-C)

0 = no help	Interviewee reports that no help (or perceived no help) is being received in the area
1 = low help	Interviewee reports that low help (or perceived low help) is currently received/needed in the area
2 = medium help	Interviewee reports that medium help (or perceived medium help) is currently received/needed in the area
3 = high help	Interviewee reports that high help (or perceived help) is currently received/ needed in the area
? = not known / prefer not to say	Interviewee does not know or does not want to answer

Issues to Consider (Suggested Time, 10 Minutes)

Section 2 relates to any help currently received by the person from friends and family. Section 3 refers to any help currently received from the services, and then additionally what help is needed from the services for this area. Note that CANFOR does not ask whether there are any discrepancies between help received and help needed from friends and family.

The guidance notes for rating whether low, medium, or high help are anchor points only. The score should reflect the perceived level of help reported by the interviewee; this may not correspond with logical views about what level of help is being provided.

9.9 Scoring and Interpretation (Section 4: Satisfaction – CANFOR-R and CANFOR-C)

NS = not satisfied	Overall, the person is not satisfied with the help received from services over the last month
S = satisfied	Overall, the person is satisfied with the help they have received from services during the last month
? = not known/ prefer not to say	The person does not know or does not want to answer this question

Issues to Consider (Suggested Time, 5 Minutes)

Only ask this question to the service user. Based on the answers to the previous questions in the domain, the person is asked how satisfied they are with the help they have received from services. Do not consider help received from friends and family here. This is a useful question to help summarise discussions about the need domain and to help you reach an overall need rating for the domain.

9.10 Scoring and Interpretation (Section 4: Contribution to Index Offence – All Versions)

| 0 = not at all | The staff member considers that difficulties in this area were not related to the index offence or reasons that the person was referred to the service. |
| 1 = a little | The staff member considers that difficulties in this area played a small role in the index offence or reasons why the person was referred to the service. |

(cont.)

| 2 = substantially | The staff member considers that difficulties in this area contributed substantially to the index offence or reasons why the person was referred to the service. |
| ? = not known/ prefer not to say | The staff member does not know or is not confident in answering this question. |

Issues to Consider (Suggested Time, 10 Minutes)

This question is only asked to the staff member. The purpose of this question is to highlight particular difficulties that may be related to future relapse or recidivism and therefore be of particular importance to target or monitor in care and treatment planning.

Additionally, the accommodation question includes a question about unreasonable delays in transfer to alternative placements (whether other inpatient services or community placements). The issue of what constitutes an unreasonable delay should be discussed and agreed upon according to local protocols.

9.11 Vignettes 1, 2, and 3 – Rating Needs Using the CANFOR-S

- Read the short vignette.
- Identify the needs according to the service user and the needs according to the staff member separately.
- Discuss whether the need domains included should be considered no need, a met need, an unmet need, or whether they should be scored as not applicable or not known.
- Consider where service user and staff views differ and consider how you might go about addressing these discrepancies.

9.12 Role-Play (Using Vignette 4) and Completion of Summary Score Sheet

- Split into pairs.
- Practice with the first five need domains on the CANFOR-R.
- Swap roles so that the interviewer then role-plays being the service user and vice versa.
- Go through the next five CANFOR-R domains.
- Discuss ratings, interview style, and issues raised with the broader group. Focus on challenges encountered and problem-solving approaches adopted to complete need ratings.

- Split back into pairs, repeating the processes above.

Practice Vignettes

Three pairs of short vignettes are provided to describe the needs of a person from a selection of the 25 CANFOR domains. These should be scored using the CANFOR-S assessment. A fourth full vignette is also included to provide a role-play for trainees; it should be scored using the CANFOR-R scale and/or associated summary score sheets.

Each vignette highlights a service user's view of their needs and the corresponding staff member's view of the needs of that service user. Suggested ratings for need domains are provided, along with a brief explanation of how and why the score was reached.

Vignette 1

Interview with Tom – A Service User

Tom has been an inpatient in a high-security hospital for three years. He doesn't think he needs to be in high security anymore and wants to be moved to a lower-security unit. He has told staff this, but they are not interested and don't seem to be doing anything about it, which annoys him. He has a diagnosis of schizophrenia and has consented to take anti-psychotic medication. This seems to be helping with his thoughts, and he reports taking some additional medication to help with any side effects. He reports no other physical health problems.

Prior to his index offence, arson, he says he drank quite a lot, but he doesn't really see this as a problem and doesn't see why he should have to go to alcohol awareness classes, especially since he can't drink in the hospital anyway. He attends different activities about four times a week but would like to do more, as he tends to get really bored and lonely when he's stuck on the ward, and he would like the opportunity to socialise more with others. He also attends education classes for help with his dyslexia, which he finds beneficial, and his primary nurse helps him read and write letters when he asks for help. He is currently seeing a therapist regarding his arson offence, which he says is OK, but he doesn't see himself as being at risk of doing this again.

Interview with Sandy – Care Coordinator for Tom

Sandy has tried to get Tom to go to alcohol awareness classes for months now, as she reports that he continues to have considerable problems in this area, but without success. She has also spent a lot of time trying to discuss this with Tom, but to no avail. He is seeing a psychologist regarding this index offence of arson, and she thinks that this seems to be helping him. But due to the nature of his offence, she doesn't think he will be transferred to a lower-security unit for some time yet, despite Tom insisting that he doesn't need to be there. He has a structured programme covering four afternoons a week, which she thinks is adequate, as he seems to like spending time by himself, away from other people. She also reports that he attends education classes twice a week for specialised help with dyslexia, and she helps him read and write letters whenever he asks her for help. She says he is compliant with his medication for a schizophrenic illness, thinks that his side effects are controlled effectively with additional medication, and that, as far as she knows, he is otherwise physically healthy at the moment.

Scoring for Vignette 1

Interview with Tom (Service User)

Accommodation	Tom says that he doesn't need to be in high security anymore and that he would like to move to a lower secure unit, but the staff doesn't seem to be doing anything about it. Therefore, according to Tom, this domain is an unmet need and should be scored as U.
Alcohol	Although he reports drinking quite a lot in the past and he has been referred to alcohol awareness classes, he doesn't go because he doesn't see this as a problem at the moment. Therefore, according to Tom, this domain is no problem and should be scored as N.
Arson	Tom says that his index offence was arson, but he doesn't see himself as a risk anymore, despite him seeing a therapist about it. Therefore, according to Tom, this domain is no problem and should be scored as N. Note that he has a history of arson, so this domain cannot be scored as not applicable, and although he is receiving an intervention, he doesn't think it is a problem anymore.
Company	Tom reports being lonely and wanting more opportunities to socialise with others. Therefore, according to Tom, this domain is an unmet need and should be scored as U.
Daytime activities	Tom says that he attends structured activities several times a week but that he'd like to do more. Therefore, according to Tom, this domain is an unmet need and should be scored as U.
Education	Tom reports being dyslexic and that he is attending education classes, which he is finding useful. Also, his primary nurse helps him to read and write letters. Therefore, according to Tom, this domain is a met need and should be scored as M.
Physical health	Tom reports taking medication to help with side effects he was suffering from and no other physical health problems at the moment. Therefore, according to Tom, this domain is a met need and should be scored as M.
Psychotic symptoms	Tom reports that he has a diagnosis of schizophrenia and that the medication he takes is helping with his thoughts. Therefore, according to Tom, this domain is a met need and should be scored as M.

Interview with Sandy (Care Coordinator)

Accommodation	Sandy says that she doesn't think Tom will be transferred to a lower-security unit for some time. Therefore, according to Sandy, this domain is not applicable and should be scored as NA.
Alcohol	Sandy reports that Tom continues to have considerable problems in this area, despite her attempts to get him to go to alcohol awareness classes and discussing issues with him. Therefore, according to Sandy, this domain is an unmet need and should be scored as U.
Arson	Sandy says that Tom is seeing a therapist regarding his arson offence and that it seems to be helping him. Therefore, according to Sandy, this domain is a met need and should be scored as M.
Company	Sandy reports that Tom seems to like spending time by himself away from other people. Therefore, according to Sandy, this domain is no problem and should be scored as N.
Daytime activities	Sandy says that Tom has a structured program that she thinks is adequate at the moment. Therefore, according to Sandy, this domain is a met need and should be scored as M.
Education	Sandy reports that Tom is dyslexic and is attending education classes twice a week for specialised help with dyslexia, and that she also helps him read and write letters. Therefore, according to Sandy, this domain is a met need and should be scored as M.
Physical health	Sandy says that Tom takes medication for side effects but is otherwise physically healthy at the moment. Therefore, according to Sandy, this domain is a met need and should be scored as M.

Vignette 2

Interview with Bill – Service User

Bill came into prison six months ago and is on remand on a burglary charge. He has his own house that he says he happily shares with his partner and two young children, and he hopes to be back there after the trial next month. He reports no difficulties in his relationship with his partner. He is currently on the health care unit of the prison, as he had become very depressed and had self-harmed two weeks ago because he could not cope with being in prison, away from his family. He says he has been prescribed some medication that is helping and that he regularly sees one of the peer volunteer 'listeners' for support.

All his food is provided for him, which he says is generally OK, and he reports that he is physically well at the moment. He has facilitated access to use the telephone to talk to his family and friends, from whom he gets a lot of support.

Interview with Damien – Care Coordinator for Bill

Damien says that Bill came into the health care unit a couple of weeks ago, having self-harmed quite badly while in the general wing of the prison. He was placed on close observations for the first week but seems to have settled more now as he is taking some medication and has been able to talk to his family quite regularly on the telephone. He said that Bill had been feeling very depressed, but that he's been prescribed some medication that seems to be helping and that Bill also sees one of the peer volunteers through the 'listeners' programme in the prison on a regular basis for support.

Damien says that Bill receives all his food from the prison and that his diet is perfectly adequate. He says he isn't sure about whether Bill will be convicted of his alleged offence, so can't be sure about the accommodation issue at the moment. Damien also says he doesn't know if Bill has any difficulties with his partner, as it's not something they have discussed, but he does know that Bill's partner is looking after their children.

Scoring for Vignette 2

Interview with Bill (Service User)

Accommodation	Bill says he is on remand, but that he has his own house that he hopes to return to after the trial next month. Therefore, according to Bill, this domain is no problem and should be scored as N.
Dependents	Bill's children are staying with his partner at his house. Therefore, according to Bill, this domain is a met need and should be scored as M.
Food	All Bill's food is provided by the prison, and he says it is generally OK. Therefore, according to Bill, this domain is a met need and should be scored as M.

(cont.)

Intimate relationships	Bill reports no difficulties in his relationship with his partner. Therefore, according to Bill, this domain is no problem and should be scored as N.
Physical health	Bill says that he is physically well at the moment, and he does not report any side effects from his medication. Therefore, according to Bill, this domain is no problem and should be scored as N.
Psychological distress	Bill says that he became very depressed and that he was not able to cope with being in prison and away from his family. He said he is now taking some medication which is helping and that he regularly sees one of the peer volunteers in the prison for support. Therefore, according to Bill, this domain is a met need and should be scored as M.
Safety to self	Bill says that he self-harmed two weeks ago. As he self-harmed in the last month, this domain is automatically considered an unmet need and should be scored as U.
Digital communication	Bill says he has facilitated access to use the telephone. Therefore, at this time, this domain is a met need and should be scored as M.

Interview with Damien (Care Coordinator)

Accommodation	Damien isn't sure whether Bill will be convicted of the offence he is on remand for, so is not sure whether accommodation will be an issue or not. Therefore, according to Damien, this domain is not known and should be scored as ?.
Dependents	Damien says that Bill's children are being looked after by Bill's partner. Therefore, according to Damien, this domain is a met need and should be scored as M.
Food	Damien says that all food is provided by the prison and that it is adequate. Therefore, according to Damien, this domain is a met need and should be scored as M.
Intimate relationships	Damien hasn't discussed this area with Bill, so isn't sure if it is a problem for Bill at the moment. Therefore, according to Damien, this domain is not known and should be scored as ?.
Psychological distress	Damien says that Bill was very depressed, but that help he is

(cont.)

	receiving (medication and seeing a listener) is helping. Therefore, according to Damien, this domain is a met need and should be scored as an M.
Safety to self	Damien says that Bill self-harmed a couple of weeks ago. Therefore, this domain is automatically considered to be an unmet need and should be scored as a U, regardless of any subsequent interventions.
Digital communication	Damien says that Bill has facilitated access to use the phone. Therefore, according to Damien, this domain is a met need and should be scored as M.

Vignette 3

Interview with Jane (Service User)

Jane has been an inpatient in a secure unit for the last 18 months. She was previously in a high-security psychiatric unit and had committed an arson offence, but she says she has no problems in this area anymore. She is getting ready to move to a hostel in the local area but has been waiting for a bed there for six weeks already. She is able to use public transport by herself and is generally OK with budgeting her money by herself. She was assessed by a welfare benefits advisor a few weeks ago, so she will receive all the benefits she is entitled to when she moves to the hostel. She is physically well and reports no problems with her sleep. Despite being a little nervous about moving to the hostel, she has not felt adversely distressed. She wears a hearing aid.

Interview with Claire (Care Coordinator)

Claire says that Jane has made good progress during the last 18 months or so that she has been on the secure unit. She says that Jane committed an arson offence and had been seeing a psychologist for one-to-one sessions up until a few months ago. That reportedly went well, and no further treatment was deemed necessary. She says that Jane is waiting to move to a supported hostel placement in the community but is getting frustrated because she has been waiting for a bed there for over a month. Claire says that Jane is OK with using public transport but still tends to get a bit mixed up with timetables, so she has been going out with Jane to help her get used to it all again, as it has been several years since Jane has lived in a community setting. She says that Jane is good with her money and that she arranged for a benefits advisor to

complete a full assessment for Jane a couple of weeks ago, so she was set for her move to the community placement.

Scoring for Vignette 3

Interview with Jane (Service User)

Accommodation	Jane says she has been waiting for a bed to become available in the local hostel for six weeks now. Therefore, according to Jane, this is an unmet need (as she has been waiting more than a month) and the domain should be scored as U.
Arson	Jane says she has a history of arson but reports no problems in this area anymore. Therefore, according to Jane, this domain is no problem should be scored as N. Note here it cannot be scored as not applicable, as she has a history of arson.
Benefits	Jane reports that she has been assessed by a benefits advisor to make sure she gets all the benefits she is entitled to when she moves to the hostel. Therefore, according to Jane, this domain is a met need and should be scored as M.
Money	Jane says she is OK with budgeting her money and doesn't report receiving any help in this area. Therefore, according to Jane, this domain is no problem and should be scored as N.
Physical health	Jane says that she is physically well but that she wears a hearing aid. She reports no difficulties with this. Therefore, according to Jane, this domain is a met need and should be scored as M.
Psychological distress	Jane says that she is a bit nervous about moving to the hostel, but that this has not been affecting her adversely. Therefore, according to Jane, this domain is no problem and should be scored as N.
Transport	Jane says she can use public transport by herself. Therefore, according to Jane, this domain is no problem and should be scored as N.

Interview with Claire (Care Coordinator)

Accommodation	Claire says that Jane is waiting to move to a supported hostel but that she has been waiting for a bed to become available for over a month. Therefore, according to Claire, this domain is an unmet need (because of the unreasonable delay experienced) and should be scored as U.

(cont.)

Arson	Claire says that Jane was seeing a psychologist up until a couple of months ago concerning her arson offence, but that no further treatment was deemed necessary. Therefore, according to Claire, this domain is no problem should be scored as N.
Benefits	Claire had arranged for a complete welfare benefits check for Jane two weeks ago; this was completed. Therefore, according to Claire, this domain is a met need and should be scored as M.
Money	Claire says that Jane is good with her money. Therefore, according to Claire, this domain is no problem and should be scored as N.
Transport	Claire says that Jane gets a bit nervous using public transport and that she has been helping her with that. Therefore, according to Claire, this domain is a met need and should be scored as M.

Vignette 4

Preamble

Leslie is a 29-year-old single mother who has an index offence of assault and a long history of alcohol misuse. She is detained under a section of the Mental Health Act and has been diagnosed with schizophrenia.

Interview with Leslie (Service User)

Leslie is currently in a low secure challenging behaviour unit. She has been in the hospital for two years with an index offence of assault of a police officer. Her daughter is in care with child and family services due to Leslie's mental health problems and she has escorted leave to visit her daughter with her social worker twice a month. She reports no incidents of violence or aggression and has had no thoughts of self-harm. She admits to having had a problem with alcohol in the past and has been attending a 'booster group' on alcohol awareness issues but says that she has not misused alcohol in the last month. She denies any problems with misusing drugs. She says that she agrees and complies with her treatment plans. She denies any history of sexual offences or arson.

A place has been allocated for her at a local hostel and she has been on two one-day visits there in the last month. She admits feeling rather anxious and worried about the move at the moment, as she has a good range of friends at the hospital and good relationships with the

staff there. She is, however, attending a leavers' group in the psychology department, which provides an opportunity for general discussion and support that she finds useful. She reports no problems with reading, writing, and using the telephone or internet, but does find transport timetables difficult to navigate and understand. She has been practising these in the leavers' group and on her visits to the hostel and now feels happier with the prospect of using public transport by herself.

She cooks for other patients in the unit on a rota basis without supervision. She admits to still needing some prompting with her self-care and has to be told to tidy her living area by the staff and other patients on the unit. She reported experiencing quite bad side effects from her depot anti-psychotic medication and that she has PRN medication available to help with the unpleasant side effects. Her medication has just been changed, so she is being monitored on a weekly basis. Her care coordinator has spent some time explaining these changes to Leslie, and she feels that she is aware of her rights from previous discussions. Apart from this, she reports no problems with her physical health or with her sleep. She feels that the voices she used to hear have been helped by the medication, and she derives some comfort from the fact that she can approach staff if she becomes distressed.

She admits to having poor money management skills and has frequently gone into debt through her hospital account. She reports no other staff interventions and has had a comprehensive benefits assessment completed by her social worker as she had difficulties completing forms by herself.

She has a full and varied activity plan, meaning that she is off the unit every day, attending groups and working in the hospital shop two mornings a week. She reports having many friends and acquaintances within the hospital but very few in the community (or the hostel) and thinks this could be a problem. She has a partner on another unit but only gets to see him about once a week at irregular social events held between the inpatient units. She reports a non-existent sex life, and this along with not being able to see her partner enough are problems that need to be addressed. She has expressed her frustrations to the nursing team, but nothing further has happened.

Interview with Jan (Care Coordinator)

Leslie has been in the hospital for two years and on the low-secure unit for four months now. Her index offence was assault of a police officer, and she has a seven-year-old daughter being cared for by local child and family services that she gets to see every couple of weeks when her social worker can organise it. Alcohol was a significant factor in her index offence, and Leslie has attended several alcohol awareness groups and is currently completing a 'booster' group. Jan does not think that drugs are a problem for Leslie at this time.

Leslie has been allocated a place at a local hostel and Jan has taken her there on day visits a couple of times now. While things are moving forward with finalising the placement, Jan considers that there have been delays in the place becoming available and the discharge process occurring and that this has led to some anxieties for Jan as the wait has been three months now.

Jan thinks that Leslie remains anxious about the move, as she has a lot of friends in the hospital, but she has been tackling this, and her confusion with how to use public transport and read timetables, through a leavers' group run by the psychology department. She doesn't think that company would be a problem for Leslie at the hostel, as Leslie seems to make friends easily. Apart from the timetables, Leslie has not reported any difficulties with reading or writing and seems fine using a telephone and the Internet.

Jan says that Leslie enjoys her activity programme and that she is off the unit every day either attending groups or working in the hospital shop. She seems to have a lot of friends in the hospital and has a partner on one of the other units who she gets to see once a week or so at organised social events. Leslie is concerned about their relationship surviving after she moves into the community, and Jan has spent a number of sessions talking to her about her options and what she could potentially do. Jan does not know of any problems with Leslie's sex life, as nothing has been discussed recently.

Leslie is actively involved with activities on the unit, and she enjoys cooking for other patients, but she does need prompting with her self-care and tidying up her living area. She has a diagnosis of schizophrenia and has been having some problems with side effects from her depot injection, so has just recently changed to a different medication that is being closely monitored. Jan is not aware of Leslie having any other physical health problems at the moment.

Since Leslie's transfer to the low secure unit, there have been no incidents of violence either to herself or others. Jan says that Leslie agrees and complies with all treatments and care plans. Jan allocates time to meet with Leslie every shift and has structured sessions on budgeting money that seem to be helping Leslie a little. She has

also just had one of the social workers help complete a full benefits assessment, as Leslie had questioned the benefits she would be eligible to receive when she moves to the hostel. Leslie has no history of sexual offending but does have a past history of arson. Jan has been addressing Leslie's offending behaviours and her illness awareness in one-on-one sessions and does not think that this is a problem for her at this time, as the offending took place some time ago during a period when Leslie was quite unwell.

Explanation of Scoring for Vignette 4

1. Examples of Scoring from the Interview with Leslie

Scoring a domain as no problem	Leslie reports being able to cook without supervision and does not think this is a problem for her. Therefore, according to Leslie, this domain is not a problem and should therefore be scored as N.
Scoring a domain as a met need	Leslie is on a low-security unit with a placement allocated at a local hostel. She has been attending a leavers' group to help address her concerns about moving on, in addition to having been on day visits to the hostel. As a place has been allocated and she reports finding the leavers' group useful, a met need is indicated. Therefore, according to Leslie, this domain should be scored as M.
Scoring a domain as an unmet need	Despite raising her frustrations about only having limited access to see her partner and having a non-existent sex life, she feels that nothing is being done to address the problem. The weekly meetings and irregular social events are not considered sufficient. This indicates an unmet need from Leslie's perspective; therefore, this domain should be scored as U. Another example of an unmet need, according to Leslie, is that she frequently goes into debt and reports no help or interventions with this.
Scoring a domain as not applicable	Leslie denies any history or current risk of sexual offending or arson. Therefore, according to Leslie, these two domains are not applicable and should be scored as NA.

2. Examples of Scoring from the Interview with Jan

Scoring a domain as no problem	Jan reports that Leslie has a prior arson offence, but she does not think that this area is a problem for her at this time. Therefore, according to Jan, this domain is no problem and should be scored as N.

(cont.)

	Other examples of domains that should be scored as no problem, from Jan's perspective, include that there have been no reported incidents of self-harm or violence in the last month.
Scoring a domain as a met need	Jan reports providing structured sessions on budgeting money that she feels are helping Leslie. Therefore, according to Jan, this domain is a met need and should be scored as M. Other examples of a met need include that Jan reports that Leslie needs a bit of prompting with her self-care and with keeping her living area clean and tidy.
Scoring a domain as an unmet need	Jan reports that although a placement at a local hostel has been found, she feels that there have been delays (in this case, three months) waiting for a bed to become available. Therefore, according to Jan, this domain is an unmet need and should be scored as U.
Scoring a domain as not applicable	Jan reports that Leslie has no history of sexual offending. Therefore, this domain is considered not applicable and should be scored as NA.
Scoring a domain as not known	Jan reports not knowing whether Leslie is experiencing any problems with her sex life, as Leslie has not spoken about this area recently. Therefore, according to Jan, this domain is not known and should be scored as ?.

Discrepancies between Ratings

Although it appears that Leslie and Jan agree on most of the areas of need, there are some differences between their responses. A notable discrepancy is the arson domain. Leslie reports no history of arson so, from her perspective, the domain is scored as not applicable (NA). However, Jan said that Leslie had a history of arson. While Jan didn't consider there to be any problems in this area at the present time, from her perspective, the domain would be scored as no problem (N) and not scored as not applicable due to the history of problems in this area.

This example highlights the real importance of assessing and recording service user and staff views separately. There could be a number of reasons why this discrepancy came about. These could include that Leslie misinterpreted the question or did not feel comfortable enough to admit to her previous offences. It is also possible that Jan was misinformed or confusing her with someone else. It could be that, in practice, some further careful questioning of both Leslie and Jan could help reveal some of these issues and therefore produce a more accurate, fully informed need rating. Whatever the reason, any discrepancies highlighted during the assessment process can be very informative points of discussion between the person and their care coordinator.

Frequently Asked Questions

Can I use the CANFOR in my service?

CANFOR was designed for use in all forensic mental health services. The CANFOR scales are therefore considered suitable to be used in secure psychiatric facilities, community forensic mental health services, probation services, and prison services.

What client groups can I use the CANFOR with?

The CANFOR was developed for use with forensic mental health service users. Other versions are available for use with adults with severe and/or enduring mental health problems (CAN), older adults (CANE), adults with developmental and intellectual disabilities (CANDID), pregnant women, and mothers (CAN-M) and emergency relief situations (HESPER).

Is the CANFOR valid and reliable?

Yes. A journal article describing the psychometric properties of the CANFOR was published in the International Journal of Methods in Psychiatric Research in 2008 (see Appendix 5). Here are the details:

Thomas, S.D.M., Slade, M., McCrone, P., Harty, M. A., Parrott, J., Thornicroft, G., & Leese, M. (2008). The reliability and validity of the forensic Camberwell Assessment of Need (CANFOR): A needs assessment for forensic mental health service users. *International Journal of Methods in Psychiatric Research, 17,* 111–120. https://doi.org/10.1002/mpr.235

What is the CANFOR-R?

The CANFOR-R is the full research version of the CANFOR (see Appendix 1). It is a semi-structured interview schedule, assessing need in 25 domains of the person's life that is suitable for research purposes.

Need domains cover a range of psychological, social, clinical, and functional areas, reflecting the broad range of needs a person can have. The CANFOR-R records the presence or absence of needs in each domain, along with details about levels of informal help received, formal help received and needed, overall satisfaction with help received from services, and whether problems/difficulties in the domains may have contributed to the index offence/reasons for referral to the service. Summary score sheets are available to help record the CANFOR-R scores (see Appendix 4).

What is the CANFOR-C?

The CANFOR-C is the full clinical version of the CANFOR (see Appendix 2). It is a semi-structured interview schedule assessing need in 25 domains of the person's life that is suitable for clinical use. Need domains cover a range of psychological, social, clinical, and functional areas, reflecting the broad range of needs a person can have. The CANFOR-C records the presence or absence of needs in each domain, along with details about levels of informal help received, formal help received and needed, and overall satisfaction with help received from services. Space is provided at the bottom of each domain page to note a summary of proposed interventions for any problems/difficulties identified and record appropriate and agreed review procedures. Summary score sheets are available to help record the CANFOR-C scores (see Appendix 4).

What is the CANFOR-S?

The CANFOR-S is a short, one-page summary of the need domains. It summarises the need rating for each domain, along with whether problems/difficulties in the domains may have contributed to the index offence/ reason for referral to the service (see Appendix 3). Experience suggests that this is the preferred and most commonly used variant of the CANFOR scales, both for research and clinical applications.

Which version of the CANFOR should I use?

Experience suggests that the CANFOR-S has the most utility in routine clinical use as well as in research. The total number of needs and number of unmet needs are the scores most commonly reported in research findings.

Why has the need rating score been changed?

We have changed how the need rating is recorded, as we found in practice that the numeric scoring in the original scales led to confusion when the assessments were being completed and interpreted. The application of the CANFOR scales remains identical, but you now record an 'N' for no need, 'M' for met need, 'U' for unmet need, 'NA' for not applicable, and '?' for not known. This revised approach is consistent with other updated CAN variants (e.g. Slade & Thornicroft, 2020).

Is there any difference between scoring a need domain as 'not applicable' (indicated by 'NA') and 'no problem' (indicated by 'N')?

A not applicable rating is only available for 5 of the 25 CANFOR domains. This additional 'not applicable' response was thought pertinent for particular domains of CANFOR where historical information may help assist in the management of the person, or where particular domains may not be applicable by virtue of the person's current situation/placement. For example, a score of not applicable in the sexual offences domain would mean that the person did not currently have any problems in this area and that they had no previous history of sexual offences. However, scoring this domain as no problem (indicated by the letter 'N') would indicate that while this domain is not currently a problem for the person, they do have a history of sexual offences. Similarly, if the person is an inpatient/prisoner and is not likely to be discharged/released in the near future (i.e. the next 6–12 months), then while it is not necessarily the case that accommodation is not a need for the person, it is likely that the need is not applicable at this time by virtue of their situation.

What if problems are identified in a particular domain for which there are no suitable interventions available locally?

The local availability of particular interventions or supports should not be used to determine the existence of a particular need. If a need exists for which there are no appropriate service interventions available, the domain should be recorded as an unmet need (indicated by the letter 'U'). It is increasingly acknowledged that forensic mental health service users often present with complex needs that cannot be met by one service. Unmet needs in particular domains may indicate the need for a multi-agency approach or collaboration, or the need to recruit workers with expertise in particular areas.

How should an item be scored if the interviewee is not confident about their answer?

If the interviewee is not confident about an answer to a particular question, then their response should be recorded as not known (indicated by '?').

What if the person refuses to answer a particular question?

If the interviewee refuses to answer a particular question or indicates that they do not want to answer it, their response should be recorded as not known (indicated by '?'). Several of the need domains cover more personal and sensitive areas, so care needs to be taken when opening discussions about them. To help, it can be beneficial to indicate at the start of the interview that some of the domains covered in the interview cover personal and potentially sensitive issues and that it is OK to not answer anything they do not feel comfortable with.

What do you do if a need doesn't exist because of a previous intervention in the past?

CANFOR ratings should only be based on any help that has been provided in the last month only. If there is an existing intervention that is helping, the domain should be rated as a met need (indicated by the letter 'M'), but if no interventions have been received during the previous month, the domain should be rated as no need (indicated by the letter 'N'). A common example of this scoring option happens in the 'Information' domain. The person may have received sufficient information in the past so that there are now no problems in the area. As such, if there is no ongoing intervention (such as sessions discussing difficulties in this area with their care coordinator), the domain should be rated as no need (indicated by the letter 'N'). Conversely, if interventions and supports have been continuing over the last month, then this domain should be scored as a met need (indicated by the letter 'M') – providing that they are deemed to be helpful.

How do you rate the over-provision of help?

The CANFOR does not routinely assess the over-provision of help. If a service is being provided in an area where the interviewee does not perceive there to be a problem, the domain would be rated as no need (indicated by the letter 'N'). However, that being said, section 3 of each domain of the CANFOR-R and CANFOR-C do record potential discrepancies between the amount or type of help being received from services and the amount or type of help that is needed (e.g. a high level of help is being provided but it is considered that a medium or low level of help is needed).

What is meant by an 'unreasonable delay' in terms of providing alternative accommodation (CANFOR need domain 1)?

A certain value judgment needs to be made when rating this particular area. During the development of the CANFOR and its testing phase, the authors chose any time that exceeded one month to be an unreasonable delay in terms of being transferred to another unit/service. If an unreasonable delay is evident, according to locally determined definitions, the accommodation domain should be scored as an unmet need (indicated by the letter 'U').

How do you interpret the overall CANFOR assessment if several of the need domains are scored as not known (indicated by '?')?

When used clinically, it may be possible to seek information about the missing domains by interviewing a range of people about the person's needs. For research purposes, it is suggested that the total need score is pro-rated according to the number of missing domain responses.

What is the difference between a met need and an unmet need?

A met need indicates that effective help is being received for problems/difficulties that have been identified in the domain area. By contrast, an unmet need indicates that either no help is currently being received for problems/difficulties identified in the domain area or that any help being received (no matter how significant or intensive) is deemed ineffective.

How do I score a need domain if the interviewee reports that there are still serious problems in the area despite receiving help?

The need rating should indicate an unmet need (U).

In the CANFOR-R and CANFOR-C, how do I rate section 3 if a service has been offered but the person has refused it?

The rating for this part of section 3 of each of the CANFOR domains relates to actual help that is being received from services. Therefore, if a support or intervention has been offered but has not been taken up, the first part of the question (level of help received) should be scored as no help (indicated by N), as no help is actually being received. Further details can be gleaned from the second part of the question (level of help needed) and also inferred through recording whether the person is satisfied with the help they have been receiving over the last month in section 4 of the domain.

How are need ratings calculated?

- The total number of met needs are calculated by adding up the number of domains where an M has been recorded; this can range from 0 to 25.
- The total number of unmet needs are calculated by adding up the number of domains where a U has been recorded; this can range from 0 to 25.
- The total number of needs are calculated by adding up the number of Ms and the number of Us recorded; this can range from 0 to 25. By way of example, if the person has six Ms and two Us recorded in their assessment (i.e. six met needs and two unmet needs), then the total number of needs is eight.

How long does it take to complete a CANFOR assessment?

The full versions of the CANFOR (the CANFOR-R and CANFOR-C) take around 20–25 minutes to complete (per interviewee). The short version (CANFOR-S) takes up to 15 minutes to complete. Staff interviews tend to be shorter in duration; the total time taken with all three CANFOR variants will shorten with practice and increased familiarity with the assessment. It is recommended that case file notes are at hand during staff interviews for quick referral, if necessary, for staff members to clarify their answers to questions.

Can I add additional need domains to CANFOR?

You can add additional individual need domains to CANFOR when you use it, but their validity and reliability would need to be established separately. Additionally, if you choose to use additional questions, it is recommended that you report them separately from the standard CANFOR domains.

Can I delete or amend domains on the CANFOR assessments?

No, do not delete or amend any existing need domains.

How do I cite the CANFOR?

Cite the 2nd edition of the CANFOR book (due to minor amendments to wording and coverage of CANFOR domains – Dependents and Digital Communication) and the 2008 article published in the *International Journal of Methods in Psychiatric Research* that outlines the psychometric properties of CANFOR. The preferred references are as follows:

Thomas, S.D.M., & Slade, M. (2021). *Camberwell Assessment of Need Forensic Version,* 2nd ed. Cambridge: Cambridge University Press.

Thomas, S.D.M., Slade, M., McCrone, P., Harty, M. A., Parrott, J., Thornicroft, G., & Leese, M. (2008). The reliability and validity of the forensic Camberwell Assessment of Need (CANFOR): A needs assessment for forensic mental health service users. *International Journal of Methods in Psychiatric Research, 17,* 111–120. https://doi.org/10.1002/mpr.235

Can I translate CANFOR into other languages?

Yes, the authors encourage such collaborations and would be keen to hear from colleagues who are interested in discussing possible translations. Please contact the lead author, Professor Stuart Thomas, for further details on translations that have been completed and ideas for new translations.

How does this book differ from the 1st edition of the CANFOR book published in 2003?

This 2nd edition includes updated details about the use of the CANFOR since its original publication (Thomas et al., 2003) and updates two of the need domains to better reflect contemporary needs and nomenclature.

Do you need any formal training in order to be able to use the CANFOR assessments?

The CANFOR was developed so that no formal training was required. It is suitable for use by a range of health professionals (such as psychiatric nurses, psychologists, and social workers) and researchers who have had some experience of clinical practice and of interviewing people who are experiencing mental illness. Some suggested training materials are provided in this book; these can be used as the basis of locally arranged in-house training. Completion of the vignettes provided will also help familiarise interviewers with the processes and decision-making involved.

What if our team would like to receive training or consultation with an external expert?

Please contact the lead author, Professor Stuart Thomas, for further details.

Do we need permission to use the CANFOR?

The CANFOR is copyrighted. There is no need to request permission or a license for any clinical, education, or research use of the CANFOR scales, providing

1. No changes to the content are made other than formatting for local use, and
2. No profit is made from it.

All versions of the CANFOR are freely available as downloads through a new dedicated section of the Research into Recovery website (http://researchintorecovery.com/can), hosted by the University of Nottingham in the UK.

What should I do if my question has not been answered here?

Please contact the lead author, Professor Stuart Thomas, in the first instance.

Appendix 1

Camberwell Assessment of Need Forensic Research Version (CANFOR-R), 2nd Edition

How to Use CANFOR-R
What Is CANFOR-R?

The CANFOR-R is a semi-structured interview schedule assessing need in 25 domains of the person's life, suitable for research purposes. Domains cover a range of psychological, social, clinical, and functional needs, reflecting the broad range of needs a person can have. Each domain is structured in the same way and is self-contained, thereby allowing for breaks to be taken during the interview as necessary.

Suggested Questioning Process for Each Domain of the CANFOR-R

1. Historically, has there been a problem/have there been any difficulties in this particular area?
2. Has this been the case over the last month?
3. Do they need any help for these problems/difficulties at the moment?
4. Are they receiving any help (informal or formal) at the moment?
5. Is any help that they are receiving actually helping and, if so, how much?
6. (*For service user interviews*) Would they say that they are satisfied with the help that they are receiving at the moment for this particular problem? Or (*For staff interviews*) did problems in this domain contribute to the index offence or reasons for referral to the service?

The first question introduces the interviewee to the general domain area. The second question then focuses the discussion on problems and difficulties experienced in the area during the time frame of interest (i.e. the past month only). The third and fourth questions seek to determine the extent of any current problems experienced and to enquire about any help that is currently being received for these difficulties. The fifth question determines the perceived effectiveness of the current help received and should then go on to enquire about any discrepancies between what is currently being received and what help is currently needed. The sixth question seeks to summarise the discussions about the domain and should inform the final overall need rating for the domain.

The overall need rating for each of the 25 need domains is scored as follows:

N = no need	Indicates that the person does not have any problems/difficulties in the area (and that they are not currently receiving any help in this area).
M = met need	Indicates that the person does currently have some problems/difficulties in this area and that effective help is being received.
U = unmet need	Indicates that the person does currently have problems/difficulties in this area and either that (from the interviewee's perspective) they are not getting any help at all for these problems/difficulties, or that the help they are receiving is not helping.
NA = not applicable	This rating is only available for five of the 25 CANFOR domains. For the sexual offending and arson domains, a not applicable score can be recorded if the interviewee reports that the person has no history of problems in the area and that they do not present a current risk in the area. Accommodation can be scored as not applicable if the person is currently an inpatient or prisoner and is not likely to be considered for transfer or discharge in the next 6–12 months. Transport

(cont.)

	can be scored as not applicable according to the same criteria. Dependents can be scored as not applicable if the interviewee reports that the person has no children or dependents.
? = not known	Indicates that the interviewee does not know about the particular domain, is not confident in their response, or does not wish to disclose any information about any problems/difficulties they might know about.

Scoring options for Sections 2, 3, and 4 of each of the CANFOR-R domains are based on the anchor points provided. While it is good practice to ask about help being received and needed, it is not necessary to complete these sections if the overall need rating for the domain no need (N). The same applies if the domain is scored as not applicable (NA) or not known (?).

Note: All versions of the CANFOR are freely available as downloads through a new dedicated section of the Research into Recovery website (http://researchintorecovery.com/can), hosted by the University of Nottingham, England.

1 Accommodation

Does the person have an appropriate place to live now or following discharge?

CAN0101   CAN0102

Do you have a place to live when you leave hospital?
Is your current accommodation placement appropriate (if in community)?

Rating	Meaning	Example
N	No problem	Living independently
M	No/moderate problem due to help given	Adequate and appropriate supported placement available
U	Serious problem	No appropriate placement identified, or available placement inappropriate, or unreasonable delays
NA	Not applicable	if not considering at present
?	Not known/prefer not to say	

If rated N, NA, or ? go to the next page

How much help with accommodation does the person receive from friends or relatives?

CAN0103   CAN0104

Rating	Meaning	Example
0	None	
1	Low help	General advice and support
2	Moderate help	Would provide help with improving accommodation, redecoration or providing furniture
3	High help	Offer place to live if own accommodation is unsatisfactory
?	Not known/prefer not to say	

How much help with accommodation does the person *receive* from local services?

CAN0105   CAN0106

How much help with accommodation does the person *need* from local services?

CAN0107   CAN0108

Rating	Meaning	Example
0	None	
1	Low help	General advice and support
2	Moderate help	Referral to housing agency for independent living
3	High help	Arranging specialist/staffed placement
?	Not known/prefer not to say	

Overall, is the person satisfied with the amount of help they are receiving with accommodation?

CAN0109

(NS=Not satisfied; S=Satisfied; ?=Not known)

In your judgement how much did problems in this area contribute to the index offence/reason for referral to the service?

CAN0110

(0=Not at all; 1=A little; 2 =Substantially; ?=Not known)

If in your judgement there is an unreasonable delay in provision of placement, give number of weeks delayed (state reason for delay)_____

CAN0111

WKS

2 Food

Does the person have difficulty in buying and preparing food?

CAN0201 CAN0202

Are you able to prepare your own meals and do your own shopping for food?

Rating	Meaning	Example
N	No problem	Able to buy and prepare meals
M	No/moderate problem due to help given	Requires prompting, supervision or assistance to buy or prepare food, or receives regular meals
U	Serious problem	Unable to buy or prepare food or not receiving adequate or appropriate help
?	Not known/prefer not to say	

If rated N or ? go to the next page

How much help does the person receive from friends or relatives with getting enough to eat?

CAN0203 CAN0204

Rating	Meaning	Example
0	None	
1	Low help	Meals provided weekly or less
2	Moderate help	Weekly help with shopping or meals provided more than weekly but not daily
3	High help	Meals provided daily (including culturally appropriate food)
?	Not known/prefer not to say	

How much help does the person *receive* from local services with buying and preparing food?

CAN0205 CAN0206

How much help does the person *need* from local services with buying and preparing food?

CAN0207 CAN0208

Rating	Meaning	Example
0	None	
1	Low help	Needs occasional prompting or assistance
2	Moderate help	Regular cooking groups, or prompting on a regular but not daily basis
3	High help	Needs meals provided daily (including culturally appropriate food)
?	Not known/prefer not to say	

Overall, is the person satisfied with the amount of help they are receiving with buying and preparing food?

CAN0209

(NS=Not satisfied; S=Satisfied; ?=Not known)

3 Looking after the Living Environment

Assessments

	Service user rating	Staff rating

Does the person have difficulty looking after their living environment?

CAN0301 CAN0302

Are you able to look after your room or home? Does anyone help you?

Rating	Meaning	Example
N	No problem	Keeps room/home clean and tidy
M	No/moderate problem due to help given	Would have difficulty maintaining cleanliness of room/home without help
U	Serious problem	Area is dirty and a potential health hazard (regardless of interventions)
?	Not known/prefer not to say	

If rated N or ? go to the next page

How much help does the person receive from friends or relatives with looking after their living environment?

CAN0303 CAN0304

Rating	Meaning	Example
0	None	
1	Low help	Prompts or helps tidy up or clean occasionally
2	Moderate help	Prompts or helps clean at least once a week
3	High help	All washing and cleaning done for the person
?	Not known/prefer not to say	

How much help does the person *receive* from local services with looking after their living environment?

CAN0305 CAN0306

How much help does the person *need* from local services with looking after their living environment?

CAN0307 CAN0308

Rating	Meaning	Example
0	None	
1	Low help	Occasional prompting or assistance by staff
2	Moderate help	Prompts or assistance at least once per week
3	High help	Majority of household tasks done by staff
?	Not known/prefer not to say	

Overall, is the person satisfied with the amount of help they are receiving in looking after their living environment?

CAN0309

(NS=Not satisfied; S=Satisfied; ?=Not known)

4 Self-care

Assessments
Service user Staff
rating   rating

Does the person have difficulty with self-care?

Do you have problems keeping yourself clean and tidy?
Does anyone remind you?

CAN0401   CAN0402

Rating	Meaning	Example
N	No problem	Untidy, but basically clean
M	No/moderate problem due to help given	Needs and gets help with self-care
U	Serious problem	Poor personal hygiene (regardless of interventions)
?	Not known/prefer not to say	

If rated N or ? go to the next page

How much help does the person receive from friends or relatives with their self-care?

CAN0403   CAN0404

Rating	Meaning	Example
0	None	
1	Low help	Occasionally prompt the person to change their clothes
2	Moderate help	Run the bath/shower or regular prompting
3	High help	Provide daily assistance with several aspects of care
?	Not known/prefer not to say	

How much help does the person *receive* from local services with their self-care?

CAN0405   CAN0406

How much help does the person *need* from local services with their self-care?

CAN0407   CAN0408

Rating	Meaning	Example
0	None	
1	Low help	Occasional prompting
2	Moderate help	Supervise weekly washing
3	High help	Supervise several aspects of self-care, self-care skills programme
?	Not known/prefer not to say	

Overall, is the person satisfied with the amount of help they are receiving with self-care?

CAN0409

(NS=Not satisfied; S=Satisfied; ?=Not known)

5 Daytime activities

Does the person have difficulty with regular, appropriate daytime activities?

CAN0501   CAN0502

How do you spend your day? Do you have a structured programme?
Do you have enough to do? (include occupation, training and higher education)

Rating	Meaning	Example
N	No problem	Able to occupy self, so no structured programme needed
M	No/moderate problem due to help given	Structured programme provided and adequate
U	Serious problem	No appropriate daytime activities offered or provided (or programme provided not appropriate/sufficient)
?	Not known/prefer not to say	

If rated N or ? go to the next page

How much help does the person receive from friends or relatives in finding or maintaining regular and appropriate daytime activities?

CAN0503   CAN0504

Rating	Meaning	Example
0	None	
1	Low help	Occasional advice about daytime activities
2	Moderate help	Participating in leisure activities with person
3	High help	Daily help with arranging daytime activities
?	Not known/prefer not to say	

How much help does the person *receive* from local services in finding or keeping regular, appropriate daytime activities?

CAN0505   CAN0506

How much help does the person *need* from local services in finding or keeping regular, appropriate daytime activities?

CAN0507   CAN0508

Rating	Meaning	Example
0	None	
1	Low help	Advice and information about activities and local facilities
2	Moderate help	Daytime activities arranged 2 or more days per week by staff
3	High help	All daytime activities arranged by staff
?	Not known/prefer not to say	

Overall, is the person satisfied with the amount of help they are receiving with daytime activities?

CAN0509

(NS=Not satisfied; S=Satisfied; ?=Not known)

In your judgement how much did problems in this area contribute to the index offence/reason for referral to the service

CAN0510

(0=Not at all; 1=A little; 2 =Substantially; ?=Not known)

6 Physical Health

Does the person have any physical disability or any physical illness?

How well do you feel physically? Are you getting any treatment for physical problems from your doctor? What about side-effects of your medication? Do you have any problems with your sleep?

CAN0601   CAN0602

Rating	Meaning	Example
N	No problem	Physically well
M	No/moderate problem due to help given	Physical ailments, such as high blood pressure, receiving appropriate treatment
U	Serious problem	Untreated physical ailments, including side-effects, or ineffective treatment
?	Not known/prefer not to say	

If rated N or ? go to the next page

How much help does the person receive from friends or relatives for physical health problems?

CAN0603   CAN0604

Rating	Meaning	Example
0	None	
1	Low help	Advised to see doctor
2	Moderate help	Clinical team informed of physical problem
3	High help	Daily help with physical health problems
?	Not known/prefer not to say	

How much help does the person *receive* from local services for physical health problems?

CAN0605   CAN0606

How much help does the person *need* from local services for physical health problems?

CAN0607   CAN0608

Rating	Meaning	Example
0	None	
1	Low help	Given advice
2	Moderate help	Regular review/involvement of specialist medical services (e.g. dietician, GP)
3	High help	Daily help or in-patient care received
?	Not known/prefer not to say	

Overall, is the person satisfied with the amount of help they are receiving for physical problems?

CAN0609

(NS=Not satisfied; S=Satisfied; ?=Not known)

7 Psychotic Symptoms

Assessments

Service user rating   Staff rating

Does the person have any psychotic symptoms, such as delusional beliefs, hallucinations, formal thought disorder, or passivity?

Do you ever hear voices, or have problems with your thoughts?
Are you on any medication or injections? What is it/are they for?

CAN0701   CAN0702

Rating	Meaning	Example
N	No problem	No positive symptoms, not at risk from symptoms and not on medication
M	No/moderate problem due to help given	Symptoms helped by medication or other help (e.g. psychology)
U	Serious problem	Currently has symptoms or symptoms resistant to treatment
?	Not known/prefer not to say	

If rated N or ? go to the next page

How much help does the person receive from friends or relatives for these psychotic symptoms?

CAN0703   CAN0704

Rating	Meaning	Example
0	None	
1	Low help	Some advice and support
2	Moderate help	Carers involved in helping with coping strategies or medication compliance
3	High help	Constant supervision of medication, and help with coping strategies
?	Not known/prefer not to say	

How much help does the person *receive* from local services for these psychotic symptoms?

CAN0705   CAN0706

How much help does the person *need* from local services for these psychotic symptoms?

CAN0707   CAN0708

Rating	Meaning	Example
0	None	
1	Low help	Maintenance of medication, infrequent review, discussed at case conference
2	Moderate help	Regular medication review and support group, discussed at management round
3	High help	Frequent medication review and/or other treatment
?	Not known/prefer not to say	

Overall, is the person satisfied with the amount of help they are receiving for psychotic symptoms?

(NS=Not satisfied; S=Satisfied; ?=Not known)

CAN0709

In your judgement how much did problems in this area contribute to the index offence/reason for referral to the service?

(0=Not at all; 1=A little; 2 =Substantially; ?=Not known)

CAN0710

8 Information on Condition and Treatment

Assessments

	Service user rating	Staff rating

Has the person had clear verbal or written information about their condition and treatment?

CAN0801 CAN0802

Have you been given clear information about your medication, treatment, and rights under the Mental Health Act?

Rating	Meaning	Example
N	No problem	No need for information, has retained from past
M	No/moderate problem due to help given	Receiving appropriate help with information on condition and treatment
U	Serious problem	Has not received or understood adequate information
?	Not known/prefer not to say	

If rated N or ? go to the next page

How much help does the person receive from friends or relatives in obtaining such information?

CAN0803 CAN0804

Rating	Meaning	Example
0	None	
1	Low help	Has had some advice from friends or relatives
2	Moderate help	Given leaflets/factsheets or put in touch with self-help groups by friends or relatives
3	High help	Regular liaison with doctors or voluntary sector sources of information or advocacy
?	Not known/prefer not to say	

How much help does the person *receive* from local services in obtaining such information?

CAN0805 CAN0806

How much help does the person *need* from local services in obtaining such information?

CAN0807 CAN0808

Rating	Meaning	Example
0	None	
1	Low help	Brief verbal or written information on illness//treatment/rights
2	Moderate help	Informal discussion with mental health staff on a range of issues relevant to treatment
3	High help	Has been given frequent or structured sessions
?	Not known/prefer not to say	

Overall, is the person satisfied with the amount of help they are receiving in obtaining information?

CAN0809

(NS=Not satisfied; S=Satisfied; ?=Not known)

9 Psychological Distress

Does the person suffer from current psychological distress?

CAN0901   CAN0902

Have you recently felt very sad or low?
Have you felt overly anxious or frightened?

Rating	Meaning	Example
N	No problem	Occasional or mild distress
M	No/moderate problem due to help given	Needs and gets ongoing support
U	Serious problem	Distress affects life significantly (regardless of interventions)
?	Not known/prefer not to say	

If rated N or ? go to the next page

How much help does the person receive from friends or relatives for this distress?

CAN0903   CAN0904

Rating	Meaning	Example
0	None	
1	Low help	Some sympathy or support
2	Moderate help	Has opportunity at least weekly to talk about distress to friend or relative
3	High help	More than weekly support or supervision
?	Not known/prefer not to say	

How much help does the person *receive* from local services for this distress?

CAN0905   CAN0906

How much help does the person *need* from local services for this distress?

CAN0907   CAN0908

Rating	Meaning	Example
0	None	
1	Low help	Assessment of mental state or occasional support
2	Moderate help	Specific psychological or social treatment. Counselled by staff at least once a week
3	High help	Daily counselling by staff, p.r.n. medication
?	Not known/prefer not to say	

Overall, is the person satisfied with the amount of help they are receiving for this distress?

CAN0909

(NS=Not satisfied; S=Satisfied; ?=Not known)

In your judgement how much did problems in this area contribute to the index offence/reasons for referral to the service?

CAN0910

(0=Not at all; 1=A little; 2 =Substantially; ?=Not known)

10 Safety to Self

Assessments
Service user Staff
rating rating

Is the person a danger to themselves?

Do you ever have thoughts of harming yourself? Have you actually harmed yourself recently? Do you put yourself in danger in any way?

CAN1001   CAN1002

Rating	Meaning	Example
N	No problem	No suicidal thoughts or thoughts of self-harm
M	No/moderate problem due to help given	Risk monitored by staff, receiving counselling
U	Serious problem	Has expressed suicidal ideas, exposed self to danger or has self-harmed
?	Not known/prefer not to say	

If rated N or ? go to the next page

How much help does the person receive from friends or relatives to reduce the risk of self-harm?

CAN1003   CAN1004

Rating	Meaning	Example
0	None	
1	Low help	Able to contact friends or relatives if feeling unsafe
2	Moderate help	Friends or relatives are usually in contact and supportive when person is feeling unsafe
3	High help	Friends or relatives in regular contact and would inform staff if disclosed/suspected risk
?	Not known/prefer not to say	

How much help does the person *receive* from local services to reduce the risk of self-harm?

CAN1005   CAN1006

How much help does the person *need* from local services to reduce the risk of self-harm?

CAN1007   CAN1008

Rating	Meaning	Example
0	None	
1	Low help	Someone to contact when feeling unsafe
2	Moderate help	Regular supportive counselling (e.g. one-to-one)
3	High help	Specific level of observation for potential self-harm, protective bedding and/or other clothing, parole and/or placement reviewed
?	Not known/prefer not to say	

Overall, is the person satisfied with the amount of help they are receiving to reduce the risk of self-harm?

CAN1009

(NS=Not satisfied; S=Satisfied; ?=Not known)

In your judgement how much did problems in this area contribute to the index offence/reasons for referral to the service?

CAN1010

(0=Not at all; 1=A little; 2=Substantially; ?=Not known)

11 Safety to Others

Has the person been violent or displayed threatening behaviour?

Have you threatened other people or been violent?
For example, have you lost your temper, or perhaps hit someone?

CAN1101 CAN1102

Rating	Meaning	Example
N	No problem	No violence or threatening behaviour in past month
M	No/moderate problem due to help given	Receives sufficient appropriate help for this problem
U	Serious problem	Recent violence or threats
?	Not known/prefer not to say	

If rated N or ? go to the next page

How much help does the person receive from friends or relatives to reduce the risk that they might harm someone else?

CAN1103 CAN1104

Rating	Meaning	Example
0	None	
1	Low help	General advice and support about threatening behaviour
2	Moderate help	Regular support and input (more than weekly)
3	High help	Daily support and/or supervision
?	Not known/prefer not to say	

How much help does the person *receive* from local services to reduce the risk that they might harm someone else?

CAN1105 CAN1106

How much help does the person *need* from local services to reduce the risk that they might harm someone else?

CAN1107 CAN1108

Rating	Meaning	Example
0	None	
1	Low help	Occasional checks on behaviour, or assessment of mental state weekly or less, advice
2	Moderate help	Regular checks on behaviour, clinical review more than weekly or escorted parole
3	High help	Close or continuous observation, daily clinical review, psychological intervention or withdrawal of parole
?	Not known/prefer not to say	

Overall, is the person satisfied with the amount of help they are receiving to reduce the risk that he or she might harm someone else?

(NS=Not satisfied; S=Satisfied; ?=Not known)

CAN1109

In your judgement, how much did problems in this area contribute to the index offence/reasons for referral to the service?

(0=Not at all; 1=A little; 2 =Substantially; ?=Not known)

CAN1110

12 Alcohol

Does the person drink excessively, or have a problem controlling their drinking?

Do you have a problem with alcohol?

CAN1201   CAN1202

Rating	Meaning	Example
N	No problem	No problem with controlled drinking
M	No/moderate problem due to help given	At risk from alcohol abuse and receiving help
U	Serious problem	Evidence of alcohol abuse recently
?	Not known/prefer not to say	

If rated N or ? go to the next page

How much help does the person receive from friends or relatives for their drinking?

CAN1203   CAN1204

Rating	Meaning	Example
0	None	
1	Low help	Told to cut down
2	Moderate help	Advised about helping agencies
3	High help	Daily monitoring and supervision of alcohol intake
?	Not known/prefer not to say	

How much help does the person *receive* from local services for their drinking?

CAN1205   CAN1206

How much help does the person *need* from local services for their drinking?

CAN1207   CAN1208

Rating	Meaning	Example
0	None	
1	Low help	Told about risks, given leaflets
2	Moderate help	Advised of helping agencies
3	High help	Supervised withdrawal programme in hospital, attending alcohol awareness group
?	Not known/prefer not to say	

Overall, is the person satisfied with the amount of help they are receiving for their drinking?

CAN1209

(NS=Not satisfied; S=Satisfied; ?=Not known)

In your judgement, how much did problems in this area contribute to the index offence/reasons for referral to the service?

CAN1210

(0=Not at all; 1=A little; 2 =Substantially; ?=Not known)

13 Drugs

Does the person have problems with drug misuse?

CAN1301   CAN1302

Do you have a problem with drugs?

Rating	Meaning	Example
N	No problem	Not misusing drugs
M	No/moderate problem due to help given	At risk from substance misuse and receiving help
U	Serious problem	Currently misusing or dependent upon illicit or prescribed drugs
?	Not known/prefer not to say	

If rated N or ? go to the next page

How much help with drug misuse does the person receive from friends or relatives?

CAN1303   CAN1304

Rating	Meaning	Example
0	None	
1	Low help	Encouraged to reduce drug use
2	Moderate help	Advised or put in touch with helping agencies
3	High help	Supervision of drug use or reporting concerns to clinical team
?	Not known/prefer not to say	

How much help with drug misuse does the person *receive* from local services?

CAN1305   CAN1306

How much help with drug misuse does the person *need* from local services?

CAN1307   CAN1308

Rating	Meaning	Example
0	None	
1	Low help	Informed about risks, given leaflets
2	Moderate help	Given details of helping agencies
3	High help	Supervised withdrawal programme, attending substance misuse group
?	Not known/prefer not to say	

Overall, is the person satisfied with the amount of help they are receiving for drug misuse?

CAN1309

(NS=Not satisfied; S=Satisfied; ?=Not known)

In your judgement, how much did problems in this area contribute to the index offence/reason for referral to the service?

CAN1310

(0=Not at all; 1=A little; 2 =Substantially; ?=Not known)

14 Company

Does the person need help with social contact?

Are you happy with your social life?
Do you wish you had more contact with others?

CAN1401   CAN1402

Rating	Meaning	Example
N	No problem	Able to organise enough social contact, has enough friends or content with own company
M	No/moderate problem due to help given	Uses organised opportunities to socialise, single-sex and mixed-sex functions available
U	Serious problem	Frequently feels lonely and isolated (regardless of interventions)
?	Not known/prefer not to say	

If rated N or ? go to the next page

How much help with social contact does the person receive from friends or relatives?

CAN1403   CAN1404

Rating	Meaning	Example
0	None	
1	Low help	Social contact less than weekly
2	Moderate help	Social contact weekly or more often
3	High help	Social contact at least four times a week
?	Not known/prefer not to say	

How much help does the person *receive* from local services in organising social contact?

CAN1405   CAN1406

How much help does the person *need* from local services in organising social contact?

CAN1407   CAN1408

Rating	Meaning	Example
0	None	
1	Low help	Given advice about social clubs or social skills groups
2	Moderate help	Day centre or community group up to 3 times a week
3	High help	Day centre or community group 4 or more times a week, facilitate single-sex and mixed-sex activities
?	Not known/prefer not to say	

Overall, is the person satisfied with the amount of help they are receiving in organising social contact?

CAN1409

(NS=Not satisfied; S=Satisfied; ?=Not known)

In your judgement, how much did problems in this area contribute to the index offence/reason for referral to the service?

CAN1410

(0=Not at all; 1=A little; 2 =Substantially; ?=Not known)

15 Intimate relationships

Does the person have any difficulty in finding a partner or in maintaining a close relationship?

CAN1501 CAN1502

Do you have a partner?
Do you have problems in your partnership/marriage/close relationship?

Rating	Meaning	Example
N	No problem	Satisfactory relationship or happy not having partner
M	No/moderate problem due to help given	Receiving helpful advice or therapy
U	Serious problem	Wants a partner and feels not having one is a problem, or ongoing conflict in existing relationship
?	Not known/prefer not to say	

If rated N or ? go to the next page

How much help does the person receive from friends or relatives with forming and maintaining close relationships?

CAN1503 CAN1504

Rating	Meaning	Example
0	None	
1	Low help	Some emotional support
2	Moderate help	Several talks, regular support
3	High help	Intensive talks and support in coping with feelings
?	Not known/prefer not to say	

How much help does the person *receive* from local services with forming and maintaining close relationships?

CAN1505 CAN1506

How much help does the person *need* from local services with forming and maintaining close relationships?

CAN1507 CAN1508

Rating	Meaning	Example
0	None	
1	Low help	A few talks
2	Moderate help	Several talks, regular support
3	High help	Therapy, social skills training
?	Not known/prefer not to say	

Overall, is the person satisfied with the amount of help they are receiving with forming and maintaining close relationships?

CAN1509

(NS=Not satisfied; S=Satisfied; ?=Not known)

In your judgement, how much did problems in this area contribute to the index offence/reason for referral to the service?

CAN1510

(0=Not at all; 1=A little; 2 =Substantially; ?=Not known)

16 Sexual expression

Assessments
Service user Staff
rating   rating

Does the person have problems with their sex life?

Are you experiencing any difficulties with sexual matters?

CAN1601 CAN1602

Rating	Meaning	Example
N	No problem	Happy with current sex life
M	No/moderate problem due to help given	Benefiting from sexual or couple therapy/other intervention
U	Serious problem	Serious sexual difficulty, such as impotence, no access or limited access to partner
?	Not known/prefer not to say	

If rated N or ? go to the next page

How much help with problems in their sex life does the person receive from friends or relatives?

CAN1603 CAN1604

Rating	Meaning	Example
0	None	
1	Low help	Some advice
2	Moderate help	Several talks, information material, providing contraceptives, etc.
3	High help	Establish contact with counselling centres and possibly accompanying the person in going there. Consistent accessibility to talk about the problem.
?	Not known/prefer not to say	

How much help with problems in their sex life does the person *receive* from local services?

CAN1605 CAN1606

How much help with problems in their sex life does the person *need* from local services?

CAN1607 CAN1608

Rating	Meaning	Example
0	None	
1	Low help	Given information about contraception, safe sex, drug-induced impotence
2	Moderate help	Regular talks about sex, medication reviewed
3	High help	Sexual or couple therapy, medication management, appropriate access to partner facilitated
?	Not known/prefer not to say	

Overall, is the person satisfied with the amount of help they are receiving for problems in their sex life?

CAN1609

(NS=Not satisfied; S=Satisfied; ?=Not known)

17 Dependents

Does the person have any difficulty looking after dependents, such as a child aged under 18 or a dependent parent?

CAN1701   CAN1702

Do you have any dependents, e.g. children under 18?
Do you have any difficulty looking after them?

Rating	Meaning	Example
N	No problem	No problem with looking after children or other dependents
M	No/moderate problem due to help given	Difficulties with parenting and receiving help Agencies facilitating access/visits
U	Serious problem	Serious difficulty looking after dependents, dependents at risk or no access due to difficulties
NA	Not applicable	if has no dependents
?	Not known/prefer not to say	

If rated N, NA, or ? go to the next page

How much help with looking after dependents does the person receive from friends and relatives?

CAN1703   CAN1704

Rating	Meaning	Example
0	None	
1	Low help	Occasional help less than once a week
2	Moderate help	Help most days, cooperating with facilitating access
3	High help	Children/other dependents living with friends/family or relatives, accompany children on access visits
?	Not known/prefer not to say	

How much help with looking after dependents does the person *receive* from local services?

CAN1705   CAN1706

How much help with looking after dependents does the person *need* from local services?

CAN1707   CAN108

Rating	Meaning	Example
0	None	
1	Low help	Attends childcare/other day care service
2	Moderate help	Help with parenting skills, facilitating access, weekly worker visits to dependent parent
3	High help	Children in foster home or in care, organising escorts to access visits, daily/almost daily worker visits to dependent parent
?	Not known/prefer not to say	

Overall, is the person satisfied with the amount of help they are receiving with looking after dependents?

CAN1709

(NS=Not satisfied; S=Satisfied; ?=Not known)

In your judgement, how much did problems in this area contribute to the index offence/reasons for referral to the service?

CAN1710

(0 =Not at all, 1=A little; 2 =Substantially; ?=Not known)

18 Basic education

Does the person lack basic skills in numeracy and literacy?

CAN1801   CAN1802

Do you have difficulty in reading, writing, or understanding English?
Can you count your change in a shop?

Rating	Meaning	Example
N	No problem	Able to read, write, and understand English forms
M	No/moderate problem due to help given	Difficulty with reading, help being received or attending adult education
U	Serious problem	Difficulty with basic skills, lack of English fluency
?	Not known/prefer not to say	

If rated N or ? go to the next page

How much help with numeracy and literacy does the person receive from friends or relatives?

CAN1803   CAN1804

Rating	Meaning	Example
0	None	
1	Low help	Occasional help to read or fill in forms
2	Moderate help	Has put them in touch with relevant classes
3	High help	Teaches the person to read, write, count change
?	Not known/prefer not to say	

How much help with numeracy and literacy does the person *receive* from local services?

CAN1805   CAN1806

How much help with numeracy and literacy does the person *need* from local services?

CAN1807   CAN1808

Rating	Meaning	Example
0	None	
1	Low help	Help filling in forms
2	Moderate help	Given advice about classes
3	High help	Attending adult education, access to interpreter
?	Not known/prefer not to say	

Overall, is the person satisfied with the amount of help they are receiving with numeracy and literacy?

CAN1809

(NS=Not satisfied; S=Satisfied; ?=Not known)

19 Digital Communication

Does the person have any difficulty in owning or using a phone, or using online services?

CAN1901   CAN1902

Do you know how to use a telephone and online services?
Is it easy to find a telephone or online services that you can use?

Rating	Meaning	Example
N	No problem	Able to use phone and online services and has appropriate access
M	No/moderate problem due to help given	Has to request to use phone or online services, facilitated access
U	Serious problem	Lacks skills to use online services
?	Not known/prefer not to say	

If rated N or ? go to the next page

How much help with phones and using online services does the person receive from friends and relatives?

CAN1903   CAN1904

Rating	Meaning	Example
0	None	
1	Low help	Occasionally helped to use phone or access to internet
2	Moderate help	At least weekly help
3	High help	Daily help, if required
?	Not known/prefer not to say	

How much help with phones and using online services does the person *receive* from local services?

CAN1905   CAN1906

How much help with phones and using online services does the person *need* from local services?

CAN1907   CAN1908

Rating	Meaning	Example
0	None	
1	Low help	Access to phone and online services upon request
2	Moderate help	Given access to computer, provided with phonecard
3	High help	Given computer and regularly helped to use phone
?	Not known/prefer not to say	

Overall, is the person satisfied with the amount of help they are receiving with phones and using online services?

CAN1909

(NS=Not satisfied; S=Satisfied; ?=Not known)

20 Transport

Does the person have any problems using public transport?

CAN2001 CAN2002

Do you have any problems using the bus, tube, or train?
Do you get a free bus pass?

Rating	Meaning	Example
N	No problem	Able to use public transport, can read timetables or has access to car
M	No/moderate problem due to help given	Bus pass or other help provided with transport
U	Serious problem	Unable to use public transport or follow timetables
NA	Not applicable	(if not tested out)
?	Not known/prefer not to say	

If rated N, NA, or ? go to the next page

How much help with transport does the person receive from friends or relatives?

CAN2003 CAN2004

Rating	Meaning	Example
0	None	
1	Low help	Encouragement to travel
2	Moderate help	Often accompanies on public transport
3	High help	Provides transport to all appointments
?	Not known/prefer not to say	

How much help does the person *receive* from local services with transport?

CAN2005 CAN2006

How much help does the person *need* from local services with transport?

CAN2007 CAN2008

Rating	Meaning	Example
0	None	
1	Low help	Provision of bus pass
2	Moderate help	Taxi card
3	High help	Transport to appointments by ambulance, facilitate travel on public transport on leave visits
?	Not known/prefer not to say	

Overall, is the person satisfied with the amount of help they are receiving with transport?

CAN2009

(NS=Not satisfied; S=Satisfied; ?=Not known)

21 Money

Assessments

Service user Staff
rating   rating

Does the person have problems budgeting their money?

CAN2101   CAN2102

Do you have problems budgeting your money?
Do you manage to pay your bills?

Rating	Meaning	Example
N	No problem	Able to buy essential items and pay bills
M	No/moderate problem due to help given	Benefits from help with budgeting
U	Serious problem	Often has no money for essential items or bills, in debt or gambling
?	Not known/prefer not to say	

If rated N or ? go to the next page

How much help does the person receive from friends or relatives in managing their money?

CAN2103   CAN2104

Rating	Meaning	Example
0	None	
1	Low help	Occasional help sorting out household bills
2	Moderate help	Calculating weekly budget
3	High help	Complete control of finance
?	Not known/prefer not to say	

How much help does the person *receive* from local services in managing their money?

CAN2105   CAN2106

How much help does the person *need* from local services in managing their money?

CAN2107   CAN2108

Rating	Meaning	Example
0	None	
1	Low help	Occasional help with budgeting
2	Moderate help	Supervised in paying rent, given weekly spending money
3	High help	Daily handouts of cash, advised of specialist agencies
?	Not known/prefer not to say	

Overall, is the person satisfied with the amount of help they are receiving with money?

CAN2109

(NS=Not satisfied; S=Satisfied; ?=Not known)

In your judgement, how much did problems in this area contribute to the index offence/reasons for referral to the service?

CAN2110

(0=Not at all; 1=A little; 2 =Substantially; ?=Not known)

22 Benefits

Is the person definitely receiving all the benefits that they are entitled to?

CAN2201 CAN2202

Are you sure that you are getting all the money you are entitled to?

Rating	Meaning	Example
N	No problem	Receiving full entitlement of benefits
M	No/moderate problem due to help given	Receives appropriate help in claiming benefits
U	Serious problem	Not receiving full entitlement of benefits
?	Not known/prefer not to say	

If rated N or ? go to the next page

How much help does the person receive from friends or relatives in obtaining their full benefit entitlement?

CAN2203 CAN2204

Rating	Meaning	Example
0	None	
1	Low help	Occasionally asks whether person is getting any money
2	Moderate help	Has made enquiries about full entitlement
3	High help	Has helped fill in forms
?	Not known/prefer not to say	

How much help does the person *receive* from local services in obtaining the full benefit entitlement?

CAN2205 CAN2206

How much help does the person *need* from local services in obtaining the full benefit entitlement?

CAN2207 CAN2208

Rating	Meaning	Example
0	None	
1	Low help	Occasional advice about entitlements
2	Moderate help	Help with applying for extra entitlements
3	High help	Comprehensive evaluation of current entitlement
?	Not known/prefer not to say	

Overall, is the person satisfied with the amount of help they are receiving in obtaining the full benefit entitlement?

CAN2209

(NS=Not satisfied; S=Satisfied; ?=Not known)

In your judgement, how much did problems in this area contribute to the index offence/reasons for referral to the service?

CAN2210

(0=Not at all; 1=A little; 2 =Substantially; ?=Not known)

23 Treatment

Does the person agree with the treatment (medical and/ or psychological) prescribed for them?

Do you agree with the treatment prescribed for you?

CAN2301   CAN2302

Rating	Meaning	Example
N	No problem	Person agrees and complies with prescribed treatments
M	No/moderate problem due to help given	Receiving help in determining appropriate treatments (e.g. does not agree but complies)
U	Serious problem	Person does not agree with treatment and does not comply
?	Not known/prefer not to say	

If rated N or ? go to the next page

How much help does the person receive from friends or relatives in understanding and accepting the care offered ?

CAN2303   CAN2304

Rating	Meaning	Example
0	None	
1	Low help	Some advice and support
2	Moderate help	Regular discussions of symptoms and appropriate advice
3	High help	Works with team to encourage acceptance of, and compliance with, treatments
?	Not known/prefer not to say	

How much help does the person *receive* from local services to understand and accept the care offered?

CAN2305   CAN2306

How much help does the person *need* from local services to understand and accept the care offered?

CAN2307   CAN2308

Rating	Meaning	Example
0	None	
1	Low help	Basic information on treatment decisions
2	Moderate help	Several discussions on reasons for treatment need. Early warning signs of relapse agreed with person
3	High help	Regular structured sessions with mental health professional, illness awareness group, psychological input
?	Not known/prefer not to say	

Overall, is the person satisfied with the amount of help they are receiving to understand and accept treatment offered?

(NS=Not satisfied; S=Satisfied; ?=Not known)

CAN2309

In your judgement, how much did problems in this area contribute to the index offence/reasons for referral to the service?

(0=Not at all; 1=A little; 2 =Substantially; ?=Not known)

CAN2310

24 Sexual offences

Does the person present a risk of sexual offending?

CAN2401   CAN2402

Do you think you might be at risk of committing a sexual offence?

Rating	Meaning	Example
N	No problem	Has history but no current risk
M	No/moderate problem due to help given	Receiving appropriate treatment or supervision
U	Serious problem	Assessed as significant continuing risk of committing sexual offences
NA	Not applicable	If no history and no risk
?	Not known/prefer not to say	

If rated N, NA, or ? go to the next page

How much help does the person receive from friends or relatives to reduce the risk of committing sexual offences?

CAN2403   CAN2404

Rating	Meaning	Example
0	None	
1	Low help	General advice and support
2	Moderate help	Regular support and input
3	High help	Inform team if disclosed/suspected at risk
?	Not known/prefer not to say	

How much help does the person *receive* from local services to reduce the risk of committing sexual offences?

CAN2405   CAN2406

How much help does the person *need* from local services to reduce the risk of committing sexual offences?

CAN2407   CAN2408

Rating	Meaning	Example
0	None	
1	Low help	Ongoing advice/monitoring of behaviour and mental state
2	Moderate help	Specific treatments, regular reviews or escorted parole
3	High help	Specific treatment intervention, daily review of behaviour and mental state or no parole
?	Not known/prefer not to say	

Overall, is the person satisfied with the amount of help they are receiving to reduce the risk of sexual offending?

CAN2409

(NS=Not satisfied; S=Satisfied; ?=Not known)

In your judgement, how much did problems in this area contribute to the index offence/reasons for referral to the service?

CAN2410

(0=Not at all; 1=A little; 2 =Substantially; ?=Not known)

25 Arson

Is the person deemed at current or potential risk of committing arson?

CAN2501 CAN2502

Do you think you might be at risk of setting fires?

Rating	Meaning	Example
N	No problem	Has history but no current risk
M	No/moderate problem due to help given	Under supervision and review
U	Serious problem	Significant continuing risk of committing arson
NA	Not applicable	If no history and no risk
?	Not known/prefer not to say	

If rated N, NA, or ? the CANFOR is complete

How much help does the person receive from friends or relatives to reduce the risk that they might set fires?

CAN2503 CAN2504

Rating	Meaning	Example
0	None	
1	Low help	General advice and support
2	Moderate help	Regular advice and support
3	High help	Informs team of disclosed/suspected risk
?	Not known/prefer not to say	

How much help does the person *receive* from local services to reduce the risk that they might set fires?

CAN2505 CAN2506

How much help does the person *need* from local services to reduce the risk that they might set fires?

CAN2507 CAN2508

Rating	Meaning	Example
0	None	
1	Low help	Occasional discussions/review of fantasies and behaviour
2	Moderate help	Regular review of fantasies and behaviour, restricted access to lighter, only smoke in designated areas
3	High help	Intensive treatment intervention or restriction of parole/access to high-risk situations
?	Not known/prefer not to say	

Overall, is the person satisfied with the amount of help they are receiving to reduce the risk of committing arson?

CAN2509

(NS=Not satisfied; S=Satisfied; ?=Not known)

In your judgement, how much did problems in this area contribute to the index offence/reasons for referral to the service?

CAN2510

(0=Not at all; 1=A little; 2 =Substantially; ?=Not known)

Appendix 2

Camberwell Assessment of Need Forensic Clinical Version (CANFOR-C), 2nd Edition

How to Use CANFOR-C

What Is CANFOR-C?

The CANFOR-C is a semi-structured interview schedule assessing need in 25 domains of the person's life, suitable for clinical use. Domains cover a range of psychological, social, clinical, and functional needs, reflecting the broad range of needs a person can have. Each domain is structured in the same way and is self-contained, thereby allowing for breaks to be taken during the interview as necessary.

Suggested Questioning Process for Each Domain of the CANFOR-C

1. Historically, has there been a problem/have there been any difficulties in this particular area?
2. Has this been the case over the last month?
3. Do they need any help for these problems/ difficulties at the moment?
4. Are they receiving any help (informal or formal) at the moment?
5. Is any help that they are receiving actually helping and, if so, how much?
6. (*For service user interviews*) Would they say that they are satisfied with the help that they are receiving at the moment for this particular problem? Or (*For staff interviews*) did problems in this domain contribute to the index offence or reasons for referral to the service?

The first question introduces the interviewee to the general domain area. The second question then focuses the discussion on problems and difficulties experienced in the area during the time frame of interest (i.e. the past month only). The third and fourth questions seek to determine the extent of any current problems experienced and to enquire about any help that is currently being received for these difficulties. The fifth question determines the perceived effectiveness of the current help received and should then go on to enquire about any discrepancies between what is currently being received and what help is currently needed. The sixth question seeks to summarise the discussions about the domain and should inform the final overall need rating for the domain.

The overall need rating for each of the 25 need domains is scored as follows:

N = no need	Indicates that the person does not have any problems/difficulties in the area (and that they are not currently receiving any help in this area).
M = met need	Indicates that the person does currently have some problems/ difficulties in this area and that effective help is being received.
U = unmet need	Indicates that the person does currently have problems/difficulties in this area and either that (from the interviewee's perspective) they are not getting any help at all for these problems/difficulties, or that the help they are receiving is not helping.
NA = not applicable	This rating is only available for 5 of the 25 CANFOR-C domains. For the sexual offending and arson domains, a not applicable score can be recorded if the interviewee reports that the person has no history of problems in the area and that they do not present a current risk in the area. Accommodation can be scored as not applicable if the person is currently an inpatient or prisoner and is not likely to be considered for transfer or discharge in the next 6–12 months. Transport can be scored as not applicable according to the same criteria. Dependents can be scored as not applicable if the interviewee reports that the person has no children or dependents.

(cont.)

? = not known/ prefer not to say	Indicates that the interviewee does not know about the particular domain, is not confident in their response, or does not wish to disclose any information about any problems/ difficulties they might know about.

Scoring options for Sections 2, 3, and 4 of each of the CANFOR-C domains are based on the anchor points provided. While it is good practice to ask about help being received and needed, it is not necessary to complete these sections if the overall need rating for the domain no need (N). The same applies if the domain is scored as not applicable (NA) or not known (?).

At the bottom of each CANFOR-C need domain page, there are boxes providing space for notes regarding possible interventions for problems/difficulties identified, as well as space for indicating appropriate review details. Consideration should be given, where appropriate, to whether problems/difficulties in the individual domains may have contributed to the index offence or reasons why the person was referred to the service they may currently be in (or attending). Additional consideration should be given to issues pertaining to risk, proximity to family, any restrictions in place regarding movements or access, relapse signs, and noting any discrepancies between viewpoints recorded.

Note: All versions of the CANFOR are freely available as downloads through a new dedicated section of the Research into Recovery website (http://researchintorecovery.com/can), hosted by the University of Nottingham, England.

1 Accommodation

Does the person have an appropriate place to live now or following discharge?

CAN0101   CAN0102

Do you have a place to live when you leave hospital?
Is your current accommodation placement appropriate (if in community)?

Rating	Meaning	Example
N	No problem	Living independently
M	No/moderate problem due to help given	Adequate and appropriate supported placement available
U	Serious problem	No appropriate placement identified, available placement inappropriate or unreasonable delays
NA	Not applicable	if not considering at present
?	Not known/prefer not to say	

If rated N, NA, or ? go to Question 2

How much help with accommodation does the person receive from friends or relatives?

CAN0103   CAN0104

Rating	Meaning	Example
0	None	
1	Low help	General advice and support
2	Moderate help	Would provide help with improving accommodation, redecoration, or providing furniture
3	High help	Offer place to live if own accommodation is unsatisfactory
?	Not known/prefer not to say	

How much help with accommodation does the person *receive* from local services?

CAN0105   CAN0106

How much help with accommodation does the person *need* from local services?

CAN0107   CAN0108

Rating	Meaning	Example
0	None	
1	Low help	General advice and support
2	Moderate help	Referral to housing agency for independent living
3	High help	Arranging specialist/staffed placement
?	Not known/prefer not to say	

Overall, is the person satisfied with the amount of help they are receiving with accommodation?

CAN0109

(NS=Not satisfied; S=Satisfied; ?=Not known)

Planning interventions	Action points	By whom	Review date
Factors to be considered (e.g. risk, proximity to family, access to services, restrictions, relapse signs, discrepancies between views, contribution to index offence/reason for referral, unreasonable delays)			

2 Food

Does the person have difficulty in buying and preparing food?

CAN0201 CAN0202

Are you able to prepare your own meals and do your own shopping for food?

Rating	Meaning	Example
N	No problem	Able to buy and prepare meals
M	No/moderate problem due to help given	Requires prompting, supervision, or assistance to buy or prepare food, or receives regular meals
U	Serious problem	Unable to buy or prepare food or not receiving adequate or appropriate help
?	Not known/prefer not to say	

If rated N or ? go to Question 3

How much help does the person receive from friends or relatives with getting enough to eat?

CAN0203 CAN0204

Rating	Meaning	Example
0	None	
1	Low help	Meals provided weekly or less
2	Moderate help	Weekly help with shopping or meals provided more than weekly but not daily
3	High help	Meals provided daily (including culturally appropriate food)
?	Not known/prefer not to say	

How much help does the person *receive* from local services with buying and preparing food?

CAN0205 CAN0206

How much help does the person *need* from local services with buying and preparing food?

CAN0207 CAN0208

Rating	Meaning	Example
0	None	
1	Low help	Needs occasional prompting or assistance
2	Moderate help	Regular cooking groups, or prompting on a regular but not daily basis
3	High help	Needs meals provided daily (including culturally appropriate food)
?	Not known/prefer not to say	

Overall, is the person satisfied with the amount of help they are receiving with buying and preparing food?

CAN0209

(NS=Not satisfied; S=Satisfied; ?=Not known)

Planning interventions	Action points	By whom	Review date
Factors to be considered (e.g. risk, proximity to family, access to services, restrictions, relapse signs, discrepancies between views)			

3 Looking after the Living Environment

Assessments

	Service user rating	Staff rating

Does the person have difficulty looking after their living environment?

Are you able to look after your room or home? Does anyone help you?

CAN0301 CAN0302

Rating	Meaning	Example
N	No problem	Keeps room/home clean and tidy
M	No/moderate problem due to help given	Would have difficulty maintaining cleanliness of room/home without help
U	Serious problem	Area is dirty and a potential health hazard (regardless of interventions)
?	Not known/prefer not to say	

If rated N or ? go to Question 4

How much help does the person receive from friends or relatives with looking after their living environment?

CAN0303 CAN0304

Rating	Meaning	Example
0	None	
1	Low help	Prompts or helps tidy up or clean occasionally
2	Moderate help	Prompts or helps clean at least once a week
3	High help	All washing and cleaning done for the person
?	Not known/prefer not to say	

How much help does the person *receive* from local services with looking after their living environment?

CAN0305 CAN0306

How much help does the person *need* from local services with looking after their living environment?

CAN0307 CAN0308

Rating	Meaning	Example
0	None	
1	Low help	Occasional prompting or assistance by staff
2	Moderate help	Prompts or assistance at least once per week
3	High help	Majority of household tasks done by staff
?	Not known/prefer not to say	

Overall, is the person satisfied with the amount of help they are receiving in looking after their living environment?

CAN0309

(NS=Not satisfied; S=Satisfied; ?=Not known)

Planning interventions	Action points	By whom	Review date
Factors to be considered (e.g. risk, proximity to family, access to services, restrictions, relapse signs, discrepancies between views)			

4 Self-care

Assessments
Service user rating Staff rating

Does the person have difficulty with self-care?

Do you have problems keeping yourself clean and tidy?
Does anyone remind you?

CAN0401 CAN0402

Rating	Meaning	Example
N	No problem	Untidy, but basically clean
M	No/moderate problem due to help given	Needs and gets help with self-care
U	Serious problem	Poor personal hygiene (regardless of interventions)
?	Not known/prefer not to say	

If rated N or ? go to Question 5

How much help does the person receive from friends or relatives with their self-care?

CAN0403 CAN0404

Rating	Meaning	Example
0	None	
1	Low help	Occasionally prompt the person to change their clothes
2	Moderate help	Run the bath/shower or regular prompting
3	High help	Provide daily assistance with several aspects of care
?	Not known/prefer not to say	

How much help does the person *receive* from local services with their self-care?

CAN0405 CAN0406

How much help does the person *need* from local services with their self-care?

CAN0407 CAN0408

Rating	Meaning	Example
0	None	
1	Low help	Occasional prompting
2	Moderate help	Supervise weekly washing
3	High help	Supervise several aspects of self-care, self-care skills programme
?	Not known/prefer not to say	

Overall, is the person satisfied with the amount of help they are receiving with self-care?

CAN0409

(NS=Not satisfied; S=Satisfied; ?=Not known)

Planning interventions	Action points	By whom	Review date
Factors to be considered (e.g. risk, proximity to family, access to services, restrictions, relapse signs, discrepancies between views)			

5 Daytime activities

Assessments

Service user rating   Staff rating

Does the person have difficulty with regular, appropriate daytime activities?

CAN0501   CAN0502

How do you spend your day? Do you have a structured programme?
Do you have enough to do? (include occupation, training, and higher education)

Rating	Meaning	Example
N	No problem	Able to occupy self, so no structured programme needed
M	No/moderate problem due to help given	Structured programme provided and adequate
U	Serious problem	No appropriate daytime activities offered or provided (or programme provided not appropriate/sufficient)
?	Not known/prefer not to say	

If rated N or ? go to Question 6

How much help does the person receive from friends or relatives in finding or maintaining regular and appropriate daytime activities?

CAN0503   CAN0504

Rating	Meaning	Example
0	None	
1	Low help	Occasional advice about daytime activities
2	Moderate help	Participating in leisure activities with person
3	High help	Daily help with arranging daytime activities
?	Not known/prefer not to say	

How much help does the person *receive* from local services in finding or keeping regular, appropriate daytime activities?

CAN0505   CAN0506

How much help does the person *need* from local services in finding or keeping regular, appropriate daytime activities?

CAN0507   CAN0508

Rating	Meaning	Example
0	None	
1	Low help	Advice and information about activities and local facilities
2	Moderate help	Daytime activities arranged 2 or more days per week by staff
3	High help	All daytime activities arranged by staff
?	Not known/prefer not to say	

Overall, is the person satisfied with the amount of help they are receiving with daytime activities?

CAN0509

(NS=Not satisfied; S=Satisfied; ?=Not known)

Planning interventions	Action points	By whom	Review date
Factors to be considered (e.g. risk, proximity to family, access to services, restrictions, relapse signs, discrepancies between views, contribution to index offence/reason for referral)			

6 Physical Health

Assessments

Service user rating   Staff rating

Does the person have any physical disability or any physical illness?

CAN0601   CAN0602

How well do you feel physically? Are you getting any treatment for physical problems from your doctor? What about side-effects of your medication? Do you have any problems with your sleep?

Rating	Meaning	Example
N	No problem	Physically well
M	No/moderate problem due to help given	Physical ailments, such as high blood pressure, receiving appropriate treatment
U	Serious problem	Untreated physical ailments, including side-effects, or ineffective treatment
?	Not known/prefer not to say	

If rated N or ? go to Question 7

How much help does the person receive from friends or relatives for physical health problems?

CAN0603   CAN0604

Rating	Meaning	Example
0	None	
1	Low help	Advised to see doctor
2	Moderate help	Clinical team informed of physical problem
3	High help	Daily help with physical health problems
?	Not known/prefer not to say	

How much help does the person *receive* from local services for physical health problems?

CAN0605   CAN0606

How much help does the person *need* from local services for physical health problems?

CAN0607   CAN0608

Rating	Meaning	Example
0	None	
1	Low help	Given advice
2	Moderate help	Regular review/involvement of specialist medical services (e.g. dietician, GP)
3	High help	Daily help or in-patient care received
?	Not known/prefer not to say	

Overall, is the person satisfied with the amount of help they are receiving for physical health?

CAN0609

(NS=Not satisfied; S=Satisfied; ?=Not known)

Planning interventions	Action points	By whom	Review date
Factors to be considered (e.g. risk, proximity to family, access to services, restrictions, relapse signs, discrepancies between views)			

7 Psychotic symptoms

Assessments

Service user rating   Staff rating

Does the person have any psychotic symptoms, such as delusional beliefs, hallucinations, formal thought disorder, or passivity?

CAN0701   CAN0702

Do you ever hear voices, or have problems with your thoughts?
Are you on any medication or injections? What is it/are they for?

Rating	Meaning	Example
N	No problem	No positive symptoms, not at risk from symptoms and not on medication
M	No/moderate problem due to help given	Symptoms helped by medication or other help (e.g. psychology)
U	Serious problem	Currently has symptoms or symptoms resistant to treatment
?	Not known/prefer not to say	

If rated N or ? go to Question 8

How much help does the person receive from friends or relatives for these psychotic symptoms?

CAN0703   CAN0704

Rating	Meaning	Example
0	None	
1	Low help	Some advice and support
2	Moderate help	Carers involved in helping with coping strategies or medication compliance
3	High help	Constant supervision of medication, and help with coping strategies
?	Not known/prefer not to say	

How much help does the person *receive* from local services for these psychotic symptoms?

CAN0705   CAN0706

How much help does the person *need* from local services for these psychotic symptoms?

CAN0707   CAN0708

Rating	Meaning	Example
0	None	
1	Low help	Maintenance of medication, infrequent review, discussed at case conference
2	Moderate help	Regular medication review and support group, discussed at management round
3	High help	Frequent medication review and/or other treatment
?	Not known/prefer not to say	

Overall, is the person satisfied with the amount of help they are receiving for psychotic symptoms?

CAN0709

(NS=Not satisfied; S=Satisfied; ?=Not known)

Planning interventions	Action points	By whom	Review date
Factors to be considered (e.g. risk, proximity to family, access to services, restrictions, relapse signs, discrepancies between views, contribution to index offence/reason for referral)			

8 Information on Condition and Treatment

Assessments

Service user rating   Staff rating

Has the person had clear verbal or written information about their condition and treatment?

CAN0801   CAN0802

Have you been given clear information about your medication, treatment and rights under the Mental Health Act?

Rating	Meaning	Example
N	No problem	No need for information, has retained from past
M	No/moderate problem due to help given	Receiving appropriate help with information on condition and treatment
U	Serious problem	Has not received or understood adequate information
?	Not known/prefer not to say	

If rated N or ? go to Question 9

How much help does the person receive from friends or relatives in obtaining such information?

CAN0803   CAN0804

Rating	Meaning	Example
0	None	
1	Low help	Has had some advice from friends or relatives
2	Moderate help	Given leaflets/factsheets or put in touch with self-help groups by friends or relatives
3	High help	Regular liaison with doctors or voluntary sector sources of information or advocacy
?	Not known/prefer not to say	

How much help does the person *receive* from local services in obtaining such information?

CAN0805   CAN0806

How much help does the person *need* from local services in obtaining such information?

CAN0807   CAN0808

Rating	Meaning	Example
0	None	
1	Low help	Brief verbal or written information on illness//treatment/rights
2	Moderate help	Informal discussion with mental health staff on a range of issues relevant to treatment
3	High help	Has been given frequent or structured sessions
?	Not known/prefer not to say	

Overall, is the person satisfied with the amount of help they are receiving in obtaining information?

CAN0809

(NS=Not satisfied; S=Satisfied; ?=Not known)

Planning interventions	Action points	By whom	Review date
Factors to be considered (e.g. risk, proximity to family, access to services, restrictions, relapse signs, discrepancies between views)			

9 Psychological Distress

Assessments

Service user Staff
rating   rating

Does the person suffer from current psychological distress?

Have you recently felt very sad or low?
Have you felt overly anxious or frightened?

CAN0901   CAN0902

Rating	Meaning	Example
N	No problem	Occasional or mild distress
M	No/moderate problem due to help given	Needs and gets ongoing support
U	Serious problem	Distress affects life significantly (regardless of interventions)
?	Not known/prefer not to say	

If rated N or ? go to Question 10

How much help does the person receive from friends or relatives for this distress?

CAN0903   CAN0904

Rating	Meaning	Example
0	None	
1	Low help	Some sympathy or support
2	Moderate help	Has opportunity at least weekly to talk about distress to friend or relative
3	High help	More than weekly support or supervision
?	Not known/prefer not to say	

How much help does the person *receive* from local services for this distress?

CAN0905   CAN0906

How much help does the person *need* from local services for this distress?

CAN0907   CAN0908

Rating	Meaning	Example
0	None	
1	Low help	Assessment of mental state or occasional support
2	Moderate help	Specific psychological or social treatment Counselled by staff at least once a week
3	High help	Daily counselling by staff, p.r.n. medication
?	Not known/prefer not to say	

Overall, is the person satisfied with the amount of help they are receiving for this distress?

CAN0909

(NS=Not satisfied; S=Satisfied; ?=Not known)

Planning interventions	Action points	By whom	Review date
Factors to be considered (e.g. risk, proximity to family, access to services, restrictions, relapse signs, discrepancies between views, contribution to index offence/reason for referral)			

10 Safety to self

Is the person a danger to themselves?

CAN1001   CAN1002

Do you ever have thoughts of harming yourself? Have you actually harmed yourself recently? Do you put yourself in danger in any way?

Rating	Meaning	Example
N	No problem	No suicidal thoughts or thoughts of self-harm
M	No/moderate problem due to help given	Risk monitored by staff, receiving counselling
U	Serious problem	Has expressed suicidal ideas, exposed self to danger or has self-harmed
?	Not known/prefer not to say	

If rated N or ? go to Question 11

How much help does the person receive from friends or relatives to reduce the risk of self-harm?

CAN1003   CAN1004

Rating	Meaning	Example
0	None	
1	Low help	Able to contact friends or relatives if feeling unsafe
2	Moderate help	Friends or relatives are usually in contact and are likely to know if feeling unsafe
3	High help	Friends or relatives in regular contact and would inform staff if disclosed/suspected risk
?	Not known/prefer not to say	

How much help does the person *receive* from local services to reduce the risk of self-harm?

CAN1005   CAN1006

How much help does the person *need* from local services to reduce the risk of self-harm?

CAN1007   CAN1008

Rating	Meaning	Example
0	None	
1	Low help	Someone to contact when feeling unsafe
2	Moderate help	Regular supportive counselling (e.g. one-to-one)
3	High help	Specific level of observation for potential self-harm, protective bedding and/or other clothing, parole and/or placement reviewed
?	Not known/prefer not to say	

Overall, is the person satisfied with the amount of help they are receiving to reduce the risk of self-harm?

CAN1009

(NS=Not satisfied; S=Satisfied; ?=Not known)

Planning interventions	Action points	By whom	Review date
Factors to be considered (e.g. risk, proximity to family, access to services, restrictions, relapse signs, discrepancies between views, contribution to index offence/reason for referral)			

11 Safety to Others

Assessments
Service user   Staff
rating   rating

Has the person been violent or displayed threatening behaviour?

Have you threatened other people or been violent?
For example, have you lost your temper, or perhaps hit someone?

Rating	Meaning	Example
N	No problem	No violence or threatening behaviour in past month
M	No/moderate problem due to help given	Receives sufficient appropriate help for this problem
U	Serious problem	Recent violence or threats
?	Not known/prefer not to say	

If rated N or ? go to Question 12

CAN1101   CAN1102

How much help does the person receive from friends or relatives to reduce the risk that they might harm someone else?

Rating	Meaning	Example
0	None	
1	Low help	General advice and support about threatening behaviour
2	Moderate help	Regular support and input (more than weekly)
3	High help	Daily support and/or supervision
?	Not known/prefer not to say	

CAN1103   CAN1104

How much help does the person *receive* from local services to reduce the risk that they might harm someone else?

CAN1105   CAN1106

How much help does the person *need* from local services to reduce the risk that they might harm someone else?

CAN1107   CAN1108

Rating	Meaning	Example
0	None	
1	Low help	Occasional checks on behaviour, or assessment of mental state weekly or less, advice
2	Moderate help	Regular checks on behaviour, clinical review more than weekly or escorted parole
3	High help	Close or continuous observation, daily clinical review, psychological intervention or withdrawal of parole
?	Not known/prefer not to say	

Overall, is the person satisfied with the amount of help they are receiving to reduce the risk that they might harm someone else?

CAN1109

(NS=Not satisfied; S=Satisfied; ?=Not known)

Planning interventions	Action points	By whom	Review date
Factors to be considered (e.g. risk, proximity to family, access to services, restrictions, relapse signs, discrepancies between views, contribution to index offence/reason for referral)			

12 Alcohol

Assessments
Service user rating   Staff rating

Does the person drink excessively, or have a problem controlling their drinking?

CAN1201   CAN1202

Does drinking cause you any problems?
Do you wish you could cut down your drinking?

Rating	Meaning	Example
N	No problem	No problem with controlled drinking
M	No/moderate problem due to help given	At risk from alcohol abuse and receiving help
U	Serious problem	Evidence of alcohol abuse recently
?	Not known/prefer not to say	

If rated N or ? go to Question 13

How much help does the person receive from friends or relatives for their drinking?

CAN1203   CAN1204

Rating	Meaning	Example
0	None	
1	Low help	Told to cut down
2	Moderate help	Advised about helping agencies
3	High help	Daily monitoring and supervision of alcohol intake
?	Not known/prefer not to say	

How much help does the person *receive* from local services for their drinking?

CAN1205   CAN1206

How much help does the person *need* from local services for their drinking?

CAN1207   CAN1208

Rating	Meaning	Example
0	None	
1	Low help	Told about risks, given leaflets
2	Moderate help	Advised of helping agencies
3	High help	Supervised withdrawal programme in hospital, attending alcohol awareness group
?	Not known/prefer not to say	

Overall, is the person satisfied with the amount of help they are receiving for their drinking?

CAN1209

(NS=Not satisfied; S=Satisfied; ?=Not known)

Planning interventions	Action points	By whom	Review date
Factors to be considered (e.g. risk, proximity to family, access to services, restrictions, relapse signs, discrepancies between views, contribution to index offence/reason for referral)			

13 Drugs

Does the person have problems with drug misuse?

CAN1301   CAN1302

Do you have a problem with drugs?

Rating	Meaning	Example
N	No problem	Not misusing drugs
M	No/moderate problem due to help given	At risk from substance misuse and receiving help
U	Serious problem	Currently misusing or dependent upon illicit or prescribed drugs
?	Not known/prefer not to say	

If rated N or ? go to Question 14

How much help with drug misuse does the person receive from friends or relatives?

CAN1303   CAN1304

Rating	Meaning	Example
0	None	
1	Low help	Encouraged to reduce drug use
2	Moderate help	Advised or put in touch with helping agencies
3	High help	Supervision of drug use or reporting concerns to clinical team
?	Not known/prefer not to say	

How much help with drug misuse does the person *receive* from local services?

CAN1305   CAN1306

How much help with drug misuse does the person *need* from local services?

CAN1307   CAN1308

Rating	Meaning	Example
0	None	
1	Low help	Informed about risks, given leaflets
2	Moderate help	Given details of helping agencies
3	High help	Supervised withdrawal programme, attending substance misuse group
?	Not known/prefer not to say	

Overall, is the person satisfied with the amount of help they are receiving for their drug misuse?

CAN1309

(NS=Not satisfied; S=Satisfied; ?=Not known)

Planning interventions	Action points	By whom	Review date
Factors to be considered (e.g. risk, proximity to family, access to services, restrictions, relapse signs, discrepancies between views, contribution to index offence/reason for referral)			

14 Company

Does the person need help with social contact?

Are you happy with your social life?
Do you wish you had more contact with others?

CAN1401   CAN1402

Rating	Meaning	Example
N	No problem	Able to organise enough social contact, has enough friends or content with own company
M	No/moderate problem due to help given	Uses organised opportunities to socialise, single-sex, and mixed-sex functions available
U	Serious problem	Frequently feels lonely and isolated (regardless of interventions)
?	Not known/prefer not to say	

If rated N or ? go to Question 15

How much help with social contact does the person receive from friends or relatives?

CAN1403   CAN1404

Rating	Meaning	Example
0	None	
1	Low help	Social contact less than weekly
2	Moderate help	Social contact weekly or more often
3	High help	Social contact at least four times a week
?	Not known/prefer not to say	

How much help does the person *receive* from local services in organising social contact?

CAN1405   CAN1406

How much help does the person *need* from local services in organising social contact?

CAN1407   CAN1408

Rating	Meaning	Example
0	None	
1	Low help	Given advice about social clubs or social skills groups
2	Moderate help	Day centre or community group up to 3 times a week
3	High help	Day centre or community group 4 or more times a week, facilitate single-sex and mixed-sex activities
?	Not known/prefer not to say	

Overall, is the person satisfied with the amount of help they are receiving in organising social contact?

CAN1409

(NS=Not satisfied; S=Satisfied; ?=Not known)

Planning interventions	Action points	By whom	Review date
Factors to be considered (e.g. risk, proximity to family, access to services, restrictions, relapse signs, discrepancies between views, contribution to index offence/reason for referral)			

15 Intimate Relationships

Assessments
Service user   Staff
rating   rating

Does the person have any difficulty in finding a partner or in maintaining a close relationship?

CAN1501   CAN1502

Do you have a partner?
Do you have problems in your partnership/marriage/close relationship?

Rating	Meaning	Example
N	No problem	Satisfactory relationship or happy not having partner
M	No/moderate problem due to help given	Receiving helpful advice or therapy
U	Serious problem	Wants a partner and feels not having one is a problem, or ongoing conflict in existing relationship
?	Not known/prefer not to say	

If rated N or ? go to Question 16

How much help does the person receive from friends or relatives with forming and maintaining close relationships?

CAN1503   CAN1504

Rating	Meaning	Example
0	None	
1	Low help	Some emotional support
2	Moderate help	Several talks, regular support
3	High help	Intensive talks and support in coping with feelings
?	Not known/prefer not to say	

How much help does the person *receive* from local services with forming and maintaining close relationships?

CAN1505   CAN1506

How much help does the person *need* from local services with forming and maintaining close relationships?

CAN1507   CAN1508

Rating	Meaning	Example
0	None	
1	Low help	A few talks
2	Moderate help	Several talks, regular support
3	High help	Therapy, social skills training
?	Not known/prefer not to say	

Overall, is the person satisfied with the amount of help they are receiving with forming and maintaining relationships?

CAN1509

(NS=Not satisfied; S=Satisfied; ?=Not known)

Planning interventions	Action points	By whom	Review date
Factors to be considered (e.g. risk, proximity to family, access to services, restrictions, relapse signs, discrepancies between views, contribution to index offence/reason for referral)			

16 Sexual Expression

Assessments
Service user rating   Staff rating

Does the person have problems with their sex life?

Are you experiencing any difficulties with sexual matters?

CAN1601   CAN1602

Rating	Meaning	Example
N	No problem	Happy with current sex life
M	No/moderate problem due to help given	Benefiting from sexual or couple therapy/other intervention
U	Serious problem	Serious sexual difficulty, such as impotence, no access or limited access to partner
?	Not known/prefer not to say	

If rated N or ? go to Question 17

How much help with problems in their sex life does the person receive from friends or relatives?

CAN1603   CAN1604

Rating	Meaning	Example
0	None	
1	Low help	Some advice
2	Moderate help	Several talks, information material, providing contraceptives, etc.
3	High help	Establish contact with counselling centres and possibly accompanying the person in going there. Consistent accessibility to talk about the problem.
?	Not known/prefer not to say	

How much help with problems in their sex life does the person *receive* from local services?

CAN1605   CAN1606

How much help with problems in their sex life does the person *need* from local services?

CAN1607   CAN1608

Rating	Meaning	Example
0	None	
1	Low help	Given information about contraception, safe sex, drug-induced impotence
2	Moderate help	Regular talks about sex, medication reviewed
3	High help	Sexual or couple therapy, medication management, appropriate access to partner facilitated
?	Not known/prefer not to say	

Overall, is the person satisfied with the amount of help they are receiving for problems in their sex life?

(NS=Not satisfied; S=Satisfied; ?=Not known)

CAN1609

Planning interventions	Action points	By whom	Review date
Factors to be considered (e.g. risk, proximity to family, access to services, restrictions, relapse signs, discrepancies between views)			

17 Dependents

Does the person have any difficulty looking after dependents, such as a child aged under 18 or a dependent parent?

CAN1701   CAN1702

Do you have any dependents, e.g. children under 18?
Do you have any difficulty looking after them?

Rating	Meaning	Example
N	No problem	No problem with looking after children or other dependents
M	No/moderate problem due to help given	Difficulties with parenting and receiving help Agencies facilitating access/visits
U	Serious problem	Serious difficulty looking after dependents, dependents at risk or no access due to difficulties
NA	Not applicable	If has no dependents
?	Not known/prefer not to say	

If rated N, NA, or ? go to Question 18

How much help with looking after dependents does the person receive from friends and relatives?

CAN1703   CAN1704

Rating	Meaning	Example
0	None	
1	Low help	Occasional help less than once a week
2	Moderate help	Help most days, cooperating with facilitating access
3	High help	Children/other dependents living with friends/family or relatives, accompany children on access visits
?	Not known/prefer not to say	

How much help with looking after dependents does the person *receive* from local services?

CAN1705   CAN1706

How much help with looking after dependents does the person *need* from local services?

CAN1707   CAN108

Rating	Meaning	Example
0	None	
1	Low help	Attends childcare/other day care service
2	Moderate help	Help with parenting skills, facilitating access, weekly worker visits to dependent parent
3	High help	Children in foster home or in care, organising escorts to access visits daily/almost daily worker visits to dependent parent
?	Not known/prefer not to say	

Overall, is the person satisfied with the amount of help they are receiving with looking after dependents?

CAN1709

(NS=Not satisfied; S=Satisfied; ?=Not known)

Planning interventions	Action points	By whom	Review date
Factors to be considered (e.g. risk, proximity to family, access to services, restrictions, relapse signs, discrepancies between views, contribution to index offence/reason for referral)			

18 Basic education

Does the person lack basic skills in numeracy and literacy?

CAN1801   CAN1802

Do you have difficulty in reading, writing, or understanding English?
Can you count your change in a shop?

Rating	Meaning	Example
N	No problem	Able to read, write, and understand English forms
M	No/moderate problem due to help given	Difficulty with reading, help being received or attending adult education
U	Serious problem	Difficulty with basic skills, lack of English fluency
?	Not known/prefer not to say	

If rated N or ? go to Question 19

How much help with numeracy and literacy does the person receive from friends or relatives?

CAN1803   CAN1804

Rating	Meaning	Example
0	None	
1	Low help	Occasional help to read or fill in forms
2	Moderate help	Has put them in touch with relevant classes
3	High help	Teaches the person to read, write, count change
?	Not known/prefer not to say	

How much help with numeracy and literacy does the person *receive* from local services?

CAN1805   CAN1806

How much help with numeracy and literacy does the person *need* from local services?

CAN1807   CAN1808

Rating	Meaning	Example
0	None	
1	Low help	Help filling in forms
2	Moderate help	Given advice about classes
3	High help	Attending adult education, access to interpreter
?	Not known/prefer not to say	

Overall, is the person satisfied with the amount of help they are receiving with numeracy and literacy?

CAN1809

(NS=Not satisfied; S=Satisfied; ?=Not known)

Planning interventions	Action points	By whom	Review date
Factors to be considered (e.g. risk, proximity to family, access to services, restrictions, relapse signs, discrepancies between views)			

19 Digital Communication

Does the person have any difficulty in owning or using a phone, or using online services?

CAN1901 CAN1902

Do you know how to use a telephone and other online services?
Is it easy to find a telephone or online services that you can use?

Rating	Meaning	Example
N	No problem	Able to use phone and online services and has appropriate access
M	No/moderate problem due to help given	Has to request to use phone or online services, facilitated access
U	Serious problem	Lacks skills to use phone or online services
?	Not known/prefer not to say	

If rated N or ? go to Question 20

How much help with phones and using online services does the person receive from friends and relatives?

CAN1903 CAN1904

Rating	Meaning	Example
0	None	
1	Low help	Occasionally helped to use phone or access to internet only for emergencies
2	Moderate help	At least weekly help
3	High help	Daily help if required
?	Not known/prefer not to say	

How much help with phones and using online services does the person *receive* from local services?

CAN1905 CAN1906

How much help with phones and using online services does the person *need* from local services?

CAN1907 CAN1908

Rating	Meaning	Example
0	None	
1	Low help	Access to phone and online services upon request
2	Moderate help	Provided with phonecard given access to computer
3	High help	Given computer and regularly helped to use phone
?	Not known/prefer not to say	

Overall, is the person satisfied with the amount of help they are receiving with phones and using online services?

CAN1909

(NS=Not satisfied; S=Satisfied; ?=Not known)

Planning interventions	Action points	By whom	Review date
Factors to be considered (e.g. risk, proximity to family, access to services, restrictions, relapse signs, discrepancies between views)			

20 Transport

Does the person have any problems using public transport?

Do you have any problems using the bus, tube, or train?
Do you get a free bus pass?

CAN2001   CAN2002

Rating	Meaning	Example
N	No problem	Able to use public transport, can read timetables or has access to car
M	No/moderate problem due to help given	Bus pass or other help provided with transport
U	Serious problem	Unable to use public transport or follow timetables
NA	Not applicable	If not tested out
?	Not known/prefer not to say	

If rated N, NA, or ? go to Question 21

How much help with transport does the person receive from friends or relatives?

CAN2003   CAN2004

Rating	Meaning	Example
0	None	
1	Low help	Encouragement to travel
2	Moderate help	Often accompanies on public transport
3	High help	Provides transport to all appointments
?	Not known/prefer not to say	

How much help does the person *receive* from local services with transport?

CAN2005   CAN2006

How much help does the person *need* from local services with transport?

CAN2007   CAN2008

Rating	Meaning	Example
0	None	
1	Low help	Provision of bus pass
2	Moderate help	Taxi card
3	High help	Transport to appointments by ambulance, facilitate travel on public transport on leave visits
?	Not known/prefer not to say	

Overall, is the person satisfied with the amount of help they are receiving with transport?

CAN2009

(NS=Not satisfied; S=Satisfied; ?=Not known)

Planning interventions	Action points	By whom	Review date
Factors to be considered (e.g. risk, proximity to family, access to services, restrictions, relapse signs, discrepancies between views)			

21 Money

Does the person have problems budgeting their money?

CAN2101   CAN2102

Do you have any problems budgeting your money?
Do you manage to pay your bills?

Rating	Meaning	Example
N	No problem	Able to buy essential items and pay bills
M	No/moderate problem due to help given	Benefits from help with budgeting
U	Serious problem	Often has no money for essential items or bills, in debt or gambling
?	Not known/prefer not to say	

If rated N or ? go to Question 22

How much help does the person receive from friends or relatives in managing their money?

CAN2103   CAN2104

Rating	Meaning	Example
0	None	
1	Low help	Occasional help sorting out household bills
2	Moderate help	Calculating weekly budget
3	High help	Complete control of finance
?	Not known/prefer not to say	

How much help does the person *receive* from local services in managing their money?

CAN2105   CAN2106

How much help does the person *need* from local services in managing their money?

CAN2107   CAN2108

Rating	Meaning	Example
0	None	
1	Low help	Occasional help with budgeting
2	Moderate help	Supervised in paying rent, given weekly spending money
3	High help	Daily handouts of cash, advised of specialist agencies
?	Not known/prefer not to say	

Overall, is the person satisfied with the amount of help they are receiving with money?

CAN2109

(NS=Not satisfied; S=Satisfied; ?=Not known)

Planning interventions	Action points	By whom	Review date
Factors to be considered (e.g. risk, proximity to family, access to services, restrictions, relapse signs, discrepancies between views, contribution to index offence/reason for referral)			

22 Benefits

Is the person definitely receiving all the benefits that they are entitled to?

CAN2201 CAN2202

Are you sure that you are getting all the money you are entitled to?

Rating	Meaning	Example
N	No problem	Receiving full entitlement of benefits
M	No/moderate problem due to help given	Receives appropriate help in claiming benefits
U	Serious problem	Not receiving full entitlement of benefits
?	Not known/prefer not to say	

If rated N or ? go to Question 23

How much help does the person receive from friends or relatives in obtaining the full benefit entitlement?

CAN2203 CAN2204

Rating	Meaning	Example
0	None	
1	Low help	Occasionally asks whether person is getting any money
2	Moderate help	Has made enquiries about full entitlement
3	High help	Has helped fill in forms
?	Not known/prefer not to say	

How much help does the person *receive* from local services in obtaining the full benefit entitlement?

CAN2205 CAN2206

How much help does the person *need* from local services in obtaining the full benefit entitlement?

CAN2207 CAN2208

Rating	Meaning	Example
0	None	
1	Low help	Occasional advice about entitlements
2	Moderate help	Help with applying for extra entitlements
3	High help	Comprehensive evaluation of current entitlement
?	Not known/prefer not to say	

Overall, is the person satisfied with the amount of help they are receiving in obtaining the full benefit entitlement?

CAN2209

(NS=Not satisfied; S=Satisfied; ?=Not known)

Planning interventions	Action points	By whom	Review date
Factors to be considered (e.g. risk, proximity to family, access to services, restrictions, relapse signs, discrepancies between views, contribution to index offence/reason for referral)			

23 Treatment

Assessments
Service user   Staff
rating   rating

Does the person agree with the treatment (medical and/ or psychological) prescribed for them?

CAN2301   CAN2302

Do you agree with the treatment prescribed for you?

Rating	Meaning	Example
N	No problem	Person agrees and complies with prescribed treatments
M	No/moderate problem due to help given	Receiving help in determining appropriate treatments (e.g. does not agree but complies)
U	Serious problem	Person does not agree with treatment and does not comply
?	Not known/prefer not to say	

If rated N or ? go to Question 24

How much help does the person receive from friends or relatives in understanding and accepting the care offered ?

CAN2303   CAN2304

Rating	Meaning	Example
0	None	
1	Low help	Some advice and support
2	Moderate help	Regular discussions of symptoms and appropriate advice
3	High help	Works with team to encourage acceptance of, and compliance with, treatments
?	Not known/prefer not to say	

How much help does the person *receive* from local services to understand and accept the care offered?

CAN2305   CAN2306

How much help does the person *need* from local services to understand and accept the care offered?

CAN2307   CAN2308

Rating	Meaning	Example
0	None	
1	Low help	Basic information on treatment decisions
2	Moderate help	Several discussions on reasons for treatment need. Early warning signs of relapse agreed with person
3	High help	Regular structured sessions with mental health professional, illness awareness group, psychological input
?	Not known/prefer not to say	

Overall, is the person satisfied with the amount of help they are receiving to understand and accept the care offered?

CAN2309

(NS=Not satisfied; S=Satisfied; ?=Not known)

Planning interventions	Action points	By whom	Review date
Factors to be considered (e.g. risk, proximity to family, access to services, restrictions, relapse signs, discrepancies between views, contribution to index offence/reason for referral)			

24 Sexual Offences

Assessments
Service user rating   Staff rating

Does the person present a risk of sexual offending?

CAN2401   CAN2402

Do you think you might be at risk of committing a sexual offence?

Rating	Meaning	Example
N	No problem	Has history but no current risk
M	No/moderate problem due to help given	Receiving appropriate treatment or supervision
U	Serious problem	Assessed as significant continuing risk of committing sexual offences
NA	Not applicable	No history and no risk
?	Not known/prefer not to say	

If rated N, NA, or ? go to Question 25

How much help does the person receive from friends or relatives to reduce the risk of committing sexual offences?

CAN2403   CAN2404

Rating	Meaning	Example
0	None	
1	Low help	General advice and support
2	Moderate help	Regular support and input
3	High help	Inform team if disclosed/suspected at risk
?	Not known/prefer not to say	

How much help does the person *receive* from local services to reduce the risk of committing sexual offences?

CAN2405   CAN2406

How much help does the person *need* from local services to reduce the risk of committing sexual offences?

CAN2407   CAN2408

Rating	Meaning	Example
0	None	
1	Low help	Ongoing advice/monitoring of behaviour and mental state
2	Moderate help	Specific treatments, regular reviews, or escorted parole
3	High help	Specific treatment intervention, daily review of behaviour and mental state, or no parole
?	Not known/prefer not to say	

Overall, is the person satisfied with the amount of help they are receiving to reduce the risk of sexual offending?

CAN2409

(NS=Not satisfied; S=Satisfied; ?=Not known)

Planning interventions	Action points	By whom	Review date
Factors to be considered (e.g. risk, proximity to family, access to services, restrictions, relapse signs, discrepancies between views, contribution to index offence/reason for referral)			

25 Arson

Is the person deemed at current or potential risk of committing arson?

CAN2501   CAN2502

Do you think you might be at risk of setting fires?

Rating	Meaning	Example
N	No problem	Has history but no current risk
M	No/moderate problem due to help given	Under supervision and review
U	Serious problem	Significant continuing risk of committing arson
NA	Not applicable	no history/risk
?	Not known/prefer not to say	

If rated N, NA, or ? the CANFOR is complete

How much help does the person receive from friends or relatives to reduce the risk that they may set fires?

CAN2503   CAN2504

Rating	Meaning	Example
0	None	
1	Low help	General advice and support
2	Moderate help	Regular support and advice
3	High help	Informs team of disclosed/suspected risk
?	Not known/prefer not to say	

How much help does the person *receive* from local services to reduce the risk that they might set fires?

CAN2505   CAN2506

How much help does the person *need* from local services to reduce the risk that they might set fires?

CAN2507   CAN2508

Rating	Meaning	Example
0	None	
1	Low help	Occasional discussions/review of fantasies and behaviour
2	Moderate help	Regular review of fantasies and behaviour, restricted access to lighter, only smoke in designated areas
3	High help	Intensive treatment intervention or restriction of parole/ access to high-risk situations
?	Not known/prefer not to say	

Overall, is the person satisfied with the amount of help they are receiving to reduce the risk of committing arson?

CAN2509

(NS=Not satisfied; S=Satisfied; ?=Not known)

Planning interventions	Action points	By whom	Review date
Factors to be considered (e.g. risk, proximity to family, access to services, restrictions, relapse signs, discrepancies between views, contribution to index offence/reason for referral)	.		

Appendix 3

Camberwell Assessment of Need Forensic Short Version (CANFOR-S), 2nd Edition

How to Use CANFOR-S
What Is CANFOR-S?

The CANFOR-S is a semi-structured interview schedule assessing need in 25 domains of the person's life. It summarises the need rating for each domain, along with whether problems/difficulties in certain domains contributed to the index offence and/or reasons for referral to the current service. The CANFOR-S is suitable for research and routine clinical use.

Suggested Questioning Process for Each Domain on the CANFOR-S

1. During the past month, have you (*they*) had any problems in this area?
2. If no, is that because of any help you (*they*) are receiving for these problems?
3. On balance, would you say that it is still a serious problem?
4. (*For staff interviews*) Do you think that problems in this domain contributed to the index offence or reasons for referral to the service?

The overall need rating for each of the 25 need domains is scored as follows:

N = no need	Indicates that the person does not have any problems/difficulties in the area and that they are not currently receiving any help in this area.
M = met need	Indicates that the person does currently have some problems/difficulties in this area and that effective help is being received.
U = unmet need	Indicates that the person does currently have problems/difficulties in this area and either that (from the interviewee's perspective) they are not getting any help at all for these problems/difficulties, or that the help they are receiving is not helping.

(cont.)

NA = not applicable	This rating is only available for five of the 25 CANFOR-S domains. For the sexual offending and arson domains, a not applicable score can be recorded if the interviewee reports that the person has no history of problems in the area and that they do not present a current risk in the area. Accommodation can be scored as not applicable if the person is currently an inpatient or prisoner and is not likely to be considered for transfer or discharge in the next 6–12 months. Transport can be scored as not applicable according to the same criteria. Dependents can be scored as not applicable if the interviewee reports that the person has no children or dependents.
? = not known / prefer not to say	Indicates that the interviewee does not know about the particular domain, is not confident in their response, or does not wish to disclose any information about any problems/difficulties they might know about.

There are four columns. The first three allow for service user, staff member, and carer views to be recorded. The last column asks the staff member to record whether they think that difficulties in the specific domain contributed to the index offence and/or reasons for referral to the current service. This question is asked for 16 of the 25 CANFOR-S need domains, as indicated on the CANFOR-S form. For this summary assessment simply record Y (yes), N (no), or ? (don't know) for this column.

The total met needs and total unmet needs should be recorded at the bottom of the page, along with the total number of needs; the latter is calculated by adding the number of met needs and the number of unmet needs together. For example, if the assessment identifies 6 Ms and 2 Us (indicating 6 met needs and 2 unmet needs across the 25 CANFOR-S need domains), then record the number 6 in the total met needs box, 2 in the total unmet needs box, and 8 (i.e. 6 met needs + 2 unmet needs) in the total needs box.

Note: All versions of the CANFOR are freely available as downloads through a new dedicated section of the Research into Recovery website (http://researchintorecovery.com/can), hosted by the University of Nottingham, England.

Camberwell Assessment of Need – Forensic Short Version

Service User name
Date of assessment __/__/__ Initials of assessor _____

N = No problem   M= Met need   U = Unmet need
NA = Not applicable **   ? = Unmet need

Assessment number	1	2	3	Index Offence
Circle who is interviewed (U = Service User, S = Staff, C = Carer)	Service User	Staff	Carer	Y / N / ?
1. **Accommodation ** *Do you have a place to live when you leave hospital?*				
2. **Food** *Are you able to prepare your own meals and do your own shopping for food?*				/////
3. **Looking after the living environment** *Are you able to look after your room? Does anyone help you?*				
4. **Self-care** *Do you have any problems keeping yourself clean and tidy?*				/////
5. **Daytime activities** *How do you spend your day? Do you have enough to do?*				
6. **Physical health** *How well do you feel physically? What about side-effects from medication?*				/////
7. **Psychotic symptoms** *Do you hear voices or have problems with your thoughts?*				
8. **Information about condition and treatment** *Have you been given clear information about your current medication, treatment, and rights?*				/////
9. **Psychological distress** *Have you recently felt sad or low? Have you recently felt anxious or frightened?*				
10. **Safety to self** *Do you have thoughts of harming yourself? Do you put yourself in danger in any way?*				
11. **Safety to others** *Have you threatened other people or been violent? For example, have you lost your temper?*				
12. **Alcohol** *Do you have a problem with alcohol?*				
13. **Drugs** *Do you have a problem with drugs?*				
14. **Company** *Are you happy with your social life? Do you wish you had more contact with others?*				
15. **Intimate relationships** *Do you have a partner? Do you have problems with your close relationships?*				
16. **Sexual expression** *How is your sex life? Are you experiencing any difficulties with sexual matters?*				/////
17. **Dependents** *Do you have any dependents, e.g. children under 18?*				
18. **Basic education** *Do you have any difficulty in reading, writing, or understanding English?*				/////
19. **Digital communication** *Do you have a phone and access to the internet?*				/////
20. **Transport ** *Do you have any problems using the bus, train, or tube? Do you get a free bus pass?*				/////
21. **Money** *Do you have problems budgeting your money? Do you manage to pay your bills?*				
22. **Benefits** *Are you sure that you are getting all the benefits you are entitled to?*				
23. **Treatment** *Do you agree with the treatment (medical and/or psychological) prescribed?*				
24. **Sexual offences** *Do you think that you might be at risk of committing a sexual offence?*				
25. **Arson** *Do you think you might be at risk of setting fires?*				

A – Met needs (count the number of Ms in the column)				Total Yes
B – Unmet needs (count the number of Us in the column)				Scores
C – Total number of needs (add together A and B)				_____

Appendix 4

CANFOR-R and CANFOR-C Summary Score Sheets, 2nd Edition

CANFOR–R and CANFOR–C
Service User Assessment Summary

Service user name _____ Date of assessment ____ / ____ / ____

Staff name _____ Date of last review ____ / ____ / ____

Scoring options	Need Rating N, M, U, NA, ?	Informal help given 0, 1, 2, 3, ?	Formal help given 0, 1, 2, 3, ?	Formal help needed 0, 1, 2, 3, ?	Satisfied with help received? NS, S, ?
CAN box number	01	03	05	07	09
1 Accommodation **					
2 Food					
3 Living environment					
4 Self-care					
5 Daytime activities					
6 Physical health					
7 Psychotic symptoms					
8 Information					
9 Psychological distress					
10 Safety to self					
11 Safety to others					
12 Alcohol					
13 Drugs					
14 Company					
15 Intimate relationships					
16 Sexual expression					
17 Dependents **					
18 Basic education					
19 Digital communication					
20 Transport **					
21 Money					
22 Benefits					
23 Treatment					
24 Sexual offences **					
25 Arson **					
Number of met needs (Add number of Ms)					
Number of unmet needs (add number of Us)					
Total number of needs (add number of Ms and Us)					

Note. ** Next to a need domain means that it can be scored as not applicable (conditions apply)

CANFOR–R and CANFOR–C
Staff Assessment Summary Sheet

Service user name _____   Date of assessment _____ /_____ /_____

Interviewer _____   Date of last review _____ /_____/_____

Scoring options	Need Rating	Informal help given	Formal help given	Formal help needed	Contributed to index offence/ referral?	Delay in provision
	N, M, U, NA, ?	0,1,2,3,?	0,1,2,3,?	0,1,2,3,?	0, 1, 2, ?	Yes or no and weeks delayed
CAN box number	02	04	06	08	10	
1 Accommodation **						
2 Food					▨	▨
3 Living environment					▨	
4 Self-care					▨	
5 Daytime activities						
6 Physical health					▨	
7 Psychotic symptoms						
8 Information					▨	
9 Psychological distress						
10 Safety to self						
11 Safety to others						
12 Alcohol						
13 Drugs						
14 Company						
15 Intimate relationships						
16 Sexual expression					▨	
17 Dependents **					▨	
18 Basic education					▨	
19 Digital communication						
20 Transport **					▨	
21 Money						
22 Benefits						
23 Treatment						
24 Sexual offences **						
25 Arson **						
Number of met needs (add number of Ms)		▨	▨	▨	▨	
Number of unmet needs (add number of Us)		▨	▨	▨	▨	
Total number of needs (add number of Ms and Us)		▨	▨	▨	▨	
Items contributing to index offence (Number of 1s and 2s)	▨	▨	▨	▨		▨

Reasons for unreasonable delay:

Details of domains contributing to index offence/reason for referral to service:

Note. ** Next to a need domain means that it can be scored as not applicable (conditions apply).

Appendix 5

CANFOR Reliability and Validity Paper

Thomas, S.D.M., Slade, M., McCrone, P., Harty, M. A., Parrott, J., Thornicroft, G., & Leese, M. (2008). The reliability and validity of the forensic Camberwell Assessment of Need (CANFOR): A needs assessment for forensic mental health service users. *International Journal of Methods in Psychiatric Research, 17,* 111–120. https://doi.org/10.1002/mpr.235

International Journal of Methods in Psychiatric Research
Int. J. Methods Psychiatr. Res. 17(2): 111–120 (2008)
Published online 4 April 2008 in Wiley InterScience
(www.interscience.wiley.com) **DOI**: 10.1002/mpr.235

The reliability and validity of the forensic Camberwell Assessment of Need (CANFOR): a needs assessment for forensic mental health service users

STUART D.M. THOMAS,[1] MIKE SLADE,[2] PAUL MCCRONE,[3] MARI-ANNE HARTY,[2] JANET PARROTT,[4] GRAHAM THORNICROFT,[2] MORVEN LEESE[2]

1 Centre for Forensic Behavioural Science, Monash University, Victorian Institute of Forensic Mental Health, Locked Bag 10, VIC 3078, Australia
2 Health Services Research Department (Box P029), Institute of Psychiatry, King's College London, UK
3 Centre for the Economics of Mental Health (Box PO24), Health Services Research Department, Institute of Psychiatry, King's College London, UK
4 The Bracton Centre, Oxleas NHS Trust, Old Bexley Lane, Bexley, Kent, UK

Abstract

No instrument exists that measures the individual needs of forensic mental health service users (FMHSUs). The aim of this study was therefore to develop a valid and reliable individual needs assessment instrument for FMHSUs that incorporated staff and service user views and measured met and unmet needs. The Camberwell Assessment of Need was used as a template to develop CANFOR. Consensual and content validity were investigated with 50 forensic mental health professionals and 60 FMHSUs. Both were found to be satisfactory. Concurrent validity was tested using the Global Assessment of Functioning and a five-point needs scale, and again was found to be satisfactory. Reliability studies were carried out with 77 service users and 65 staff in high and medium security psychiatric services in the UK. Inter-rater reliability, rating whether a need was present or not, was high for service users (0.991) and staff (0.998). Similarly high reliability was found for unmet needs (0.985 and 0.972, respectively). Test–retest reliability was found to be moderately high for service users (0.795) and staff (0.852) when ratings were made two weeks apart. Similar levels were found for ratings of unmet needs (0.813 and 0.699, respectively). The average interview time was 23 minutes. CANFOR has good validity and reliability, and is suitable for further testing with other service user groups. Copyright © 2008 John Wiley & Sons, Ltd.

Key words: needs assessment, forensic mental health, reliability, validity, CANFOR

Background

The needs of forensic mental health service users (FMHSUs) continue be the topic of much academic and clinical debate. Coupled with this, in the UK and elsewhere, there has been continuing emphasis on the recommendation to use needs assessments as a central component in service planning, development and evaluation in order to deliver effective and efficient services (e.g. Cohen and Eastman, 2000; Department of Health and Home Office, 1992; White et al., 2006).

FMHSUs can and do have complex and multiple needs that change over time and which may well require support from a number of different services at any one time (e.g. Thomas et al., 2004; Thomas et al.,

112   *Thomas et al.*

2003). Being able to assess these needs in a standard way is therefore imperative, both for the delivery of effective treatment interventions and for the development of tailored aftercare packages. However, the means and methods of assessing the individual needs of this client group have, to some extent, been neglected with the focus instead being much more on the need to develop assessment tools focussing on security and risk issues (e.g. Collins and Davies, 2005; Maden et al., 1993; Shaw et al., 1994).

One scale that does include some need domains, the Level of Service Inventory – Revised (Andrews and Bonta, 1995), only considers criminogenic needs (i.e. needs that are associated with changes in the probability of recidivism), and omits more general (individual) needs due to their weak association with recidivism. However, the individual needs of FMHSUs also require assessment in a coherent and consistent fashion (Shaw, 2002); for a number of ethical, just, and plain decent reasons (Andrews et al., 2006). Therefore this study aimed to develop a needs assessment that specifically focussed on identifying the health and social needs of FMHSUs.

Methods

Development of CANFOR

The Camberwell Assessment of Need (CAN: Phelan et al., 1995; Slade et al., 1999) was used as a template. While many of the CAN need domains were applicable to FMHSUs, not all of their needs were represented adequately or in sufficient depth. Therefore the CAN was adapted, with questions reworded and domains added. Revisions were carried out by an interdisciplinary team, covering community and forensic services, comprised of four of the authors (GT, MH, PM and JP) and one other experienced consultant psychiatrist. The original criteria of the CAN were preserved, i.e. that it should (1) have adequate psychometric properties, (2) be valid and reliable, (3) be able to be completed within 30 minutes, (4) be usable by a wide range of professionals, (5) be easily learned and used without extensive training, (6) be suitable for routine clinical practice and research, and (7) be applicable to a wide range of populations and settings.

CANFOR, like the other CAN instruments, was developed to be able to record the views of service users and staff separately for each need domain. The scoring of each need domain is therefore based directly on the views of the interviewee. Any differences in perceptions of need (between service users and staff) are apparent by directly comparing the ratings.

A need is defined as being present when the interviewee indicates that there have been difficulties in a particular area over the last month. If a need is deemed present, the domain is then scored as either met or unmet. A met need is defined where a difficulty has been identified for which an appropriate intervention is currently being received. An unmet need is defined where a difficulty has been identified for which no interventions are currently being received, from either formal or informal sources, or that any interventions or support being received are not helping. If a need is not considered to be present it can be scored as no need or, in certain instances, not applicable. The total need score is defined as the sum of the number of met needs and unmet needs (Thomas et al., 2003).

One of the authors (MH) piloted the draft on 20 service users and 17 staff members. Based on this piloting phase, revisions were then made to CANFOR in consultation with the research team. In particular one item, originally called 'concordance', was revised to address 'treatment' needs instead.

Participants

Studies were carried out in a medium security psychiatric hospital and a high security psychiatric hospital in the UK. Initial lists of all inpatients in the hospitals on determined census dates were collated. A sample size calculation suggested that a sample of 45 service users would be sufficient to estimate the inter-rater reliability to within a confidence interval of approximately ±0.05 (i.e. from 0.9–1.00 assuming that it was about 0.9), and that a sample of 30 service users from each site would be able to estimate the test–retest reliability to within approximately ±0.1 (i.e. from 0.65 to 0.85, assuming that it was about 0.7).

A stratified random sample for each hospital unit (ward) was selected by one of the authors (ST). Half of the service users on each unit were originally selected, taking every second name on the alphabetical bed listings. Individuals were excluded if they had an intellectual disability diagnosis, or where otherwise requested by the Responsible Medical Officers or clinical teams. The latter included an inability to give informed written consent and safety issues associated with completing the interviews. On exclusion, the next person on the list was approached. Eligible participants were

Int. J. Methods Psychiatr. Res. 17(2): 111–120 (2008)
DOI: 10.1002/mpr

approached and given brief verbal and written details about the study, and then a time was arranged for the researcher to return, usually the following day, to answer any questions and to seek written consent. Their primary nurse, or a qualified member of staff who identified themselves as knowing the individual participants well, was then approached and interviewed separately. This process continued until either the requisite sample had been reached for the unit, or all of the potential participants had been approached. Ethical approval was obtained from the host institution and the Local Research Ethics Committees for the two hospitals.

Validity studies
Content validity was investigated using a brief questionnaire to assess the views of a convenience sample of FMHSUs in medium and high security psychiatric services. Participants were asked to rate each CANFOR domain for it's relevance in relation to the individual needs of FMHSUs, using a four-point scale from 'not at all relevant' to 'very relevant'; and to identify the most and least relevant domains, whether any areas of need were not covered, and any other comments they had about the measure.

Consensual validity was explored by a survey of 50 forensic mental health professionals from a range of professional backgrounds in the UK. Those surveyed were a convenience sample of experts in the field, identified by members of the research team. They were sent a brief postal questionnaire that investigated their views about the need for CANFOR, ratings of relevance, comprehensiveness and length, and whether there were any missing need domains in the measure.

Two methods of investigating face validity were used. First, the Flesch ease of reading score (Grammatik Software, 1992) was calculated to indicate how difficult it was to understand the text used in CANFOR. Second, the staff survey included questions as to the utility and comprehensiveness of CANFOR in highlighting the major needs of FMHSUs.

Due to a lack of a published 'gold standard' to compare the CANFOR with, two approaches to establishing construct validity were used. First, the Global Assessment of Functioning (GAF) Scale (APA, 1994) was scored, with separate symptoms, disability and total GAF ratings rated. Ratings on each of the subscales were made according to a continuous scale ranging from 90 down to zero, with lower scores indicating

greater severity and/or lower functioning. In this instance, GAF scores represented the most severe level of symptoms and disability observed during the last month. Second, staff rated each service users overall level of need on a five-point scale (1 = no to low, 2 = low to moderate, 3 = moderate, 4 = moderate to high, and 5 = high level of overall need). The GAF and five-point need ratings were completed before CANFOR was completed.

Reliability studies
Four raters were used to test inter-rater reliability, comprising three social science graduates and a psychiatrist. No formal training was provided. All interviews were carried out with the interviewer and a second 'silent' rater in a quiet room with the interviewee. For the reliability studies, the interview comprised an interviewer who asked to respondents (FMHSUs or staff members) the questions and rated the responses, while the second rater sat silently in the room simultaneously scoring the responses to the questions independent of the interviewer. Interviews were timed by the interviewers.

Test–retest reliability was investigated by reinterviewing half of the service users, one or two weeks after the first interview. This time frame was selected following the assumption that needs would remain relatively stable over that time period (Streiner and Norman, 1995, p. 114). The same interviewer completed both interviews.

Statistical analysis
Summary descriptive statistics were calculated. For construct validity, the association between CANFOR scores, GAF scores and estimated need level were assessed using Kendall's tau-b rank correlation coefficient. Intra-class correlations (ICCs) were calculated, using a two-way mixed model defining agreement in terms of consistency, to assess both inter-rater and test–retest reliability for continuous scores (Bland and Altman, 1986) (need versus no need and unmet need versus met or no need). The ICCs represent the ratio of the variance of the true score between subjects and the total variance (Leese et al., 2001). Analyses were carried out in the Statistical Package for Social Sciences (SPSS version 15.0, 2006). The Flesch Readability test was computed using Grammatik Software (1992) and verified using the readability statistics option in Microsoft Word.

Int. J. Methods Psychiatr. Res. 17(2): 111–120 (2008)
DOI: 10.1002/mpr

Results

Content validity

Sixty FMHSUs were interviewed. All items were thought to be at least moderately relevant. Additional items were suggested by two FMHSUs, but referred to interventions (psychotherapy and drug treatment) rather than needs.

Consensual validity

Forensic mental health professionals expressed that there was a need for such a measure and that CANFOR was relevant and useful to highlight individual need in FMHSUs. The consensus was that the instrument was adequate in length. All agreed that developing a shortened one-page version of CANFOR would be clinically useful. The only additional items suggested concerned risk-specific information, i.e. extreme levels of violence directed towards self or others. As CANFOR was developed as a screen to highlight problem areas, not to provide in-depth risk assessment and/or management data, these items were not added to the instrument.

Face validity

CANFOR had a Flesch ease of reading score of 59, which means that it is the preferred level for most readers, with an average word length of 1.63 syllables indicating that 'most readers could comprehend the vocabulary'. The general opinion of the forensic mental health professionals surveyed was that items included in CANFOR covered the major difficulties faced by FMHSUs in inpatient and community settings.

Reliability and validity study

One hundred and five FMHSUs were approached to participate in the reliability and validity sub-study. Twenty-six declined and two were excluded for safety reasons at the request of the Responsible Medical Officer. Refusers were significantly more likely than participants to be younger, male and resident in medium security psychiatric services.

The staff interviewed for this component of the study were all qualified mental health nurses, who reported having worked predominantly on the particular units and having known the individual participants for a minimum of six months (or sufficiently well where length of stay was less than six months). The characteristics of the FMHSUs are shown in Table 1.

Profile of needs

Staff rated FMHSUs as having an average of 8.7 total needs [standard deviation (SD) = 2.3] out of a possible 25, with 2.3 (SD = 1.8) of these needs considered to be unmet. A simple histogram of total need scores revealed a normal distribution (Figure 1), while total unmet need scores were positively skewed, with 63% of the sample being rated as having two or less unmet needs overall (Figure 2). Highest staff-rated needs (regardless of being met or unmet) were in the domains of daytime activities (95%), psychotic symptoms (83%) and information (77%). Highest levels of unmet need, according to staff perceptions, were in the areas of daytime activities (42%), psychotic symptoms (33%) and accommodation (26%).

By contrast, FMHSUs reported significantly less needs than staff ($t = 4.79$, $p < 0.01$), with an average of 6.8 needs (SD = 2.4) out of a possible 25. They reported that an average of 2.4 of these needs (SD = 2.1) were unmet. Needs were most commonly reported by FMHSUs in the areas of daytime activities (88%), physical health (62%) and psychotic symptoms (61%). Highest levels of unmet need were reported with accommodation (34%), daytime activities (23%) and information (25%). The distribution of total needs and unmet needs reported was consistent with the staff ratings displayed in Figures 1 and 2.

Construct validity

Total need scores on CANFOR, as rated by the primary nurse, were compared with GAF scores and the five-point need score. The GAF scale was completed for 60 of the FMHSUs and the estimated need score for the entire sample. The mean GAF symptoms score was 54.5 (SD = 21), and mean disability score of 63.9 (SD = 18.2). The mean overall need score, on the five-point scale, was 3.4 (SD = 1.04, range 1–5). The GAF total score, GAF symptoms score and ratings on the five-point needs scale followed a normal distribution. GAF disability scores were negatively skewed, with 30% of the sample being rated by primary nurses as functioning at the top end of the scale (score of 80 or higher).

Total needs were significantly associated with GAF symptom scores [$\tau = -0.27$, $N = 52$, 95% confidence interval (CI) = 0.07–0.469], GAF disability scores ($\tau = -0.24$, $N = 52$, 95% CI = 0.06–0.42) and GAF total scores ($\tau = -0.27$, $N = 52$, 95% CI = 0.07–0.46); with less severe symptoms, disability and overall functioning being associated with a lower number of overall needs.

Int. J. Methods Psychiatr. Res. 17(2): 111–120 (2008)
DOI: 10.1002/mpr

Table 1. Characteristics of the high security and medium security sample

Characteristics	High security unit n = 52 (%)	Medium security unit n = 25 (%)	Total N = 77 (%)
Gender			
Male	31 (60)	22 (88)	53 (69)
Age			
Mean	39.54	37.12	38.75
Median	37	36	36
Standard deviation	11.40	10.69	11.16
Range	22–79	21–66	21–79
Length of stay (months)			
Mean	100.78	16.44	73.04
Median	87	15	37.50
SD	104.65	10.14	94.47
Ethnicity[1]			
White	37 (71)	10 (40)	47 (61)
Other	15 (29)	15 (60)	30 (45)
Diagnosis[2]			
Schizophrenia, schizotypal and delusional disorders	37 (71)	24 (96)	61 (79)
Personality disorder	13 (25)	1 (4)	14 (18)
Mood affective disorders	2 (4)	–	2 (3)
Source of admission			
Prison	36 (69)	11 (44)	47 (61)
Medium security	11 (21)	3 (12)	14 (18)
High security	1 (2)	8 (32)	9 (12)
Other	4 (8)	3 (12)	7 (9)
Section of MHA (1983)			
Section 3	8 (15)	2 (8)	10 (13)
Section 35	1 (2)	–	1 (1)
Section 37 (inc. Notional)	4 (8)	5 (20)	9 (12)
Section 38	3 (6)	–	3 (4)
Section 37/41	26 (50)	16 (64)	42 (55)
Section 47/49	7 (14)	–	7 (9)
Section 48/49	–	1 (4)	1 (1)
CPIA (1964 or 1991)	2 (4)	1 (4)	3 (4)
Section 45a	1 (2)	–	1 (1)
Legal category (according to case files)			
Mental illness	32 (62)	24 (96)	56 (73)
Psychopathic disorder	12 (23)	–	12 (16)
Mental illness and psychopathic disorder	8 (15)	1 (4)	9 (12)
Index offence[3]			
Homicide	21 (40)	5 (20)	26 (34)
Violence	9 (17)	12 (48)	21 (27)
Sexual offence	4 (8)	3 (12)	7 (9)
Arson	9 (17)	–	9 (12)
No index offence	5 (10)	–	5 (6)
Other	4 (8)	5 (20)	9 (12)

[1] Based on self-report of patient.
[2] ICD-10 category diagnoses from case files (WHO, 1992).
[3] Where there was more than one index offence recorded the most serious offence was reported.

Int. J. Methods Psychiatr. Res. 17(2): 111–120 (2008)
DOI: 10.1002/mpr

116   *Thomas et al.*

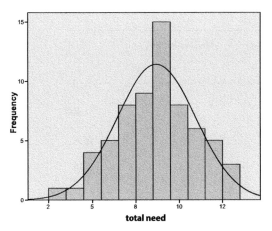

Figure 1. Histogram of total number of staff rated needs.

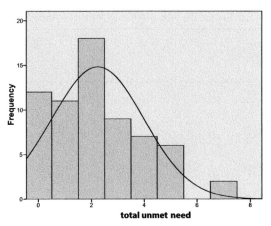

Figure 2. Histogram of total number of staff rated unmet needs.

There was a significant positive correlation between the total needs score on CANFOR and the five-point need score ($\tau = 0.37$, $N = 62$, 95% CI = 0.19–0.55).

Unmet needs were weakly associated with GAF symptom scores ($\tau = -0.210$, $N = 52$, 95% CI = -0.01–0.42), GAF disability scores ($\tau = -0.118$, $N = 52$, 95% CI = -0.03–0.324) and GAF total scores ($\tau = -0.182$, $N = 52$, 95% CI = -0.03–0.39); with higher GAF scores (showing increased levels of functional ability) being related to lower levels of unmet need. There was also a positive correlation between unmet needs and the five-point needs score ($\tau = 0.176$, $N = 62$, 95% CI = -0.01–0.37).

Reliability studies
Seventy-seven service users and 65 staff were interviewed at Time 1. Due to staffing difficulties the remaining 12 staff interviews were not completed within a timeframe that would lead to meaningful comparison.

Inter-rater reliability
Fifty-one service user and 38 staff interviews were silently rated by a second person in the room at Time 1. ICCs for total needs score and total unmet need scores indicated a high level of agreement between raters for both staff and FMHSU interviews (Table 2).

Test–retest reliability
Thirty-two FMHSUs and 32 staff were interviewed at Time 2. CANFOR data were complete for 27 of the

Table 2. Inter-rater and test–retest reliability for total CANFOR scores

Total number of needs	Intraclass correlation coefficient (ICC)	
	User rating	Staff rating
Inter-rater reliability	$n = 51$	$n = 38$
Needs, whether met or unmet	0.991	0.998
Unmet needs	0.985	0.972
Test–retest reliability	$n = 30$	$n = 27$
Needs, whether met or unmet	0.795	0.852
Unmet needs	0.813	0.699

staff and 30 of the FMHSUs re-interviewed at Time 2. ICCs for total need scores and total unmet needs were moderate to high (Table 2).

Domain specific reliability coefficients
ICCs were also calculated for each of the 25 CANFOR domains. ICCs were calculated in relation to overall agreement about the presence of a need (regardless of whether it was met or unmet) and agreement on ratings of unmet needs only for staff and FMHSU interviews separately (Tables 3 and 4).

Discussion
This study aimed to develop and test the reliability and validity of an individual needs assessment for forensic mental health service users. CANFOR was developed to highlight frequent problem areas for FMHSUs. It

Int. J. Methods Psychiatr. Res. 17(2): 111–120 (2008)
DOI: 10.1002/mpr

Table 3. Reliability of each CANFOR domain based on interviews with staff

CANFOR domains	Presence of a need		Rating an unmet need	
	Inter-rater	Test–retest	Inter-rater	Test–retest
Accommodation	0.98	0.89	0.92	0.70
Food	1	0.64	0.92	0
Living environment	1	0.78	1	0
Self care	1	0.31	1	0
Daytime activities	1	0.79	1	0.88
Physical health	0.96	0.83	0.79	0
Psychotic symptoms	1	0.95	1	0.43
Information	0.97	−0.22	1	0
Psychological distress	0.96	0.64	0.66	0
Safety to self (self-harm)	1	0.94	1	0.91
Safety to others (violence)	0.98	0.60	0.92	−0.13
Alcohol	1	0.31	0.92	−0.11
Drugs	0.98	0.68	0.92	0
Company	1	0.70	1	0.82
Intimate relationships	1	0.57	1	−0.13
Sexual expression	0.98	0.87	0.88	0.79
Childcare	1	0.68	1	1
Basic education	1	0.84	1	0
Telephone	1	1	1	0
Transport	1	0	1	0
Money	1	0.79	1	1
Benefits	0.97	0	0.80	0
Treatment	0.98	0.76	0.80	0
Sexual offences	0.95	0.82	0	1
Arson	1	0.68	–	0.79

Note: Inter-rater reliability with 38 staff, test–retest reliability with 27 staff.

does not seek to go into any detail about the identified problem domains. Where particular difficulties are identified it is recommended that further assessments are carried out to detail specific risks and the need for specialized interventions.

Validity studies
In spite of a lack of a 'gold standard' comparator at the time of development, the validity studies suggest that there is a need for an individual needs assessment for FMHSUs and that CANFOR may have some utility is this respect.

Inter-rater reliability studies
CANFOR demonstrates high levels of inter-rater reliability with both staff and service user interviews. Domain specific analyses suggested that raters agreed

least when interviewing staff about psychological distress and physical health; and about treatment and self-harm when interviewing FMHSUs. Additional attention may need to be paid to these areas when assessing needs.

Test–retest reliability
Overall, the coefficients for test–retest reliability with the FMHSU participants were moderate to high. Lowest consistency between ratings when interviewing FMHSUs at two close time intervals were found for money, physical health, sexual expression and psychotic symptoms. The lowest consistency between ratings when interviewing staff about their service users was found for violence, alcohol, intimate relationships and psychotic symptoms. Reasons for these inconsistencies are not immediately clear from the data. There has

Int. J. Methods Psychiatr. Res. 17(2): 111–120 (2008)
DOI: 10.1002/mpr

118   *Thomas et al.*

Table 4. Reliability of each CANFOR domain based on interviews with service users

CANFOR domains	Presence of a need		Rating an unmet need	
	Inter-rater	Test–retest	Inter-rater	Test–retest
Accommodation	1	0.75	1	0.55
Food	0.98	0.97	1	0
Living environment	1	−0.10	0	0
Self care	0	0	0	0
Daytime activities	0.99	0.68	0.97	0.83
Physical health	0.98	0.67	0.93	−0.07
Psychotic symptoms	1	0.79	1	0.36
Information	0.98	0.49	0.98	0.60
Psychological distress	1	0.92	1	0.87
Safety to self (self-harm)	0.91	0.34	0.84	0.62
Safety to others (violence)	0.99	0.63	0.94	0.63
Alcohol	0.80	0.66	0	0.79
Drugs	1	1	0	0
Company	0.98	0.64	0.80	0.49
Intimate relationships	1	0.79	1	0.79
Sexual expression	1	0.33	1	0.33
Childcare	0.95	0.68	0.95	0.66
Basic education	1	0.76	1	0.88
Telephone	0.97	−0.07	0.85	0
Transport	1	−0.07	1	0
Money	0.99	−0.10	0.94	−0.07
Benefits	0.96	0.85	0.96	0.52
Treatment	0.96	0.56	0.83	0
Sexual offences	0.97	1	1	0
Arson	1	0	0	0

Note: Inter-rater reliability with 51 service users, test–retest reliability with 30 service users.

been some suggestion that mood state should be taken into account when interpreting subjective measures relating to quality of life based on self-report (e.g. Holloway and Carson, 1999; Ruggeri et al., 2003). It may be that these domains are more susceptible to changes in psychopathology among the FMHSUs; hence the changes in reported need between Time 1 and Time 2. Similarly, the low consistency in certain need domains for staff interviews may be indicative of changes in presentation of the FMHSUs. Alternatively, it may be that being involved in the research simply led them to identify need areas for their patients, which they then acted upon before they were re-interviewed. Further study investigating these issues in relation to 'sensitivity to change' may therefore be indicated. This remains an area for further scientific inquiry.

In terms of making ratings as accurate and consistent as possible for both clinical and research use; some recent research has suggested that there may be differences in the perceptions of, and ratings made by, people from different professional backgrounds (Davies et al., 2006), due to differences in their clinical frames of reference, any specialist training received and levels of experience. Ecob et al. (2004) suggest the need for specialized training to address any adjustments required to counter such effects. Due to the additional complexities of FMHSUs, and addressing identified needs within the wider framework of risk and accountability (Andrews and Bonta, 2003; Cohen and Eastman, 2000), some formalized training about how to score CANFOR may address some of the differences between raters, and lead to greater consistency and therefore practical utility.

Int. J. Methods Psychiatr. Res. 17(2): 111–120 (2008)
DOI: 10.1002/mpr

CANFOR offers one potential approach to assessing the individual needs of FMHSUs in a systematic and simple way and allows comparability with other CAN assessments and populations. A book describing the three versions of CANFOR, along with a guide to training, is now available (Thomas et al., 2003), translations of the CANFOR scale are underway in several other countries including Spain and Japan, and the CAN website contains further details about CANFOR.

Further research is required to ascertain its suitability in correctional and community services, with larger samples covering wider geographical areas and different services. Further work is also warranted to examine the relationships between need, risk and outcome in the short and longer term (e.g. Andrews et al., 2006) in order that the best possible care and treatment can be provided to patients while at the same time protecting the wider community.

Acknowledgements

The authors would like to acknowledge the assistance of Jonathan Bindman in the initial revision of the CAN and Elaine Brohan for her helpful comments on an earlier draft of this paper. The authors would also like to acknowledge the Department of Health for funding this research.

Declaration of Interests

The authors have no competing interests.

References

American Psychiatric Association (APA). Diagnostic and Statistical Manual of Mental Disorders, 4th Edition (DSM-IV). Washington, DC: APA, 1994.

Andrews DA, Bonta J. The Level of Service Inventory – Revised. Toronto: Multi-Health Systems, 1995.

Andrews DA, Bonta J. The Psychology of Criminal Conduct, 3rd Edition. Cincinnati, OH: Andersen Publishing Co., 2003.

Andrews DA, Bonta J, Wormith JS. The recent past and near future of risk and/or need assessment. Crime & Delinquency 2006; 52(1): 7–27. DOI: 10.1177/0011128705281756

Bland JM, Altman DG. Statistical methods for assessing agreement between two methods of clinical assessment. Lancet 1986; 307–10.

Cohen A, Eastman N. Assessing Forensic Mental Health Need. Policy, Theory and Research. London: Gaskell, 2000.

Collins M, Davies S. The Security Needs Assessment Profile: a multidimensional approach to measuring security needs. Int J Forensic Mental Health 2005; 4(1): 39–52.

Davies JP, Heyman B, Godin PM, Shaw MP, Reynolds L. The problems of offenders with mental disorders: a plurality of perspectives within a single mental health care organisation. Soc Sci Med 2006; 63(4): 1097–108. DOI:10.1016/j.socscimed.2006.03.002

Department of Health and Home Office. Review of Health and Social Services for Mentally Disordered Offenders and Others Requiring Similar Services (The Reed Report), Final Summary Report, CM2088. London: HMSO, 1992.

Ecob R, Croudace TJ, White IR, Evans JE, Harrison GL, Sharp D, Jones PB. Multilevel investigation of variation in HoNOS ratings by mental health professionals: a naturalistic study of consecutive referrals. Int J Methods Psychiatr Res 2004; 13(3): 152–64.

Grammatik Software. Grammatik 5 for Windows version 1.0. Essex: Reference Software International, 1992.

Holloway F, Carson J. Subjective quality of life, psychopathology, satisfaction with care and insight: an exploratory study. Int J Soc Psychiatry 1999; 45(4): 259–67.

Leese MN, White IR, Schene AH, Koeter MWJ, Ruggeri M, Gaite L. Reliability in multi-site psychiatric studies. Int J Methods Psychiatr Res 2001; 10(1): 29–42.

Maden A, Curle C, Meux S, Burrow S, Gunn J. The treatment and security needs of patients in special hospitals. Criminal Behaviour and Mental Health 1993; 3: 290–306.

Phelan M, Slade M, Thornicroft G, Dunn G, Holloway F, Wykes T, Strathdee G, Loftus L, McCrone P, Hayward P. The Camberwell Assessment of Need: the validity and reliability of an instrument to assess the needs of the seriously mentally ill. Br J Psychiatry 1995; 167(5): 589–95.

Ruggeri M, Pacati P, Goldberg D. Neurotics are dissatisfied with life, but not with services. The South Verona Outcomes Project 7. General and Hospital Psychiatry 2003; 25(5): 338–44. DOI: 10.1016/S0163-8343(03)00063-X

Shaw J. Needs assessment for mentally disordered offenders is different. J Forensic Psychiatry 2002; 13(1): 14–7. DOI: 10.1080/09585180210123249

Shaw J, McKenna J, Snowdon P, Cameron B, McMahon D, Kilshaw J. The North West Region I: Clinical features and placement needs of patients detained in Special Hospitals. J Forensic Psychiatry 1994; 5(1): 93–105.

Slade M, Loftus L, Phelan M, Thornicroft G, Wykes T. The Camberwell Assessment of Need. London: Gaskell, 1999.

SPSS. Statistical Package for Social Sciences version 15.0. Chicago, IL: SPSS Inc., 2006.

Streiner DL, Norman GR. Health measurement scales. A practical guide to their development and use. Oxford: Oxford University Press, 1995, pp. 104–26.

Thomas S, Dolan M, Thornicroft G. Revisiting the need for high security psychiatric hospitals in England. J Forensic Psychiatry Psychology 2004; 15(2): 197–207. DOI: 10.1080/1478994040001703976

Int. J. Methods Psychiatr. Res. 17(2): 111–120 (2008)
DOI: 10.1002/mpr

120   *Thomas et al.*

Thomas S, Harty MA, Parrott J, McCrone P, Slade M, Thornicroft G. The Forensic CAN (CANFOR). A Needs Assessment for Forensic Mental Health Service Users. London: Gaskell, 2003.

White P, Chant D, Whiteford H. A comparison of Australian men with psychotic disorders remanded for criminal offences and a community group of psychotic men who have not offended. Aust NZ J Psychiatry 2006; 40(3): 260–5. DOI: 10.1111/j.1440-1614.2006.01783.x

World Health Organization (WHO). The ICD-10 Classification of Mental and Behavioural Disorders. Clinical Descriptions and Diagnostic Guidelines. Geneva: World Health Organization, 1992.

Correspondence: Stuart Thomas, Centre for Forensic Behavioural Science, Monash University, Victorian Institute of Forensic Mental Health, Locked Bag 10, VIC 3078, Australia.

Telephone +61 3 9495 9162

Fax +61 3 9495 9195

Email: stuart.thomas@med.monash.edu.au

Int. J. Methods Psychiatr. Res. 17(2): 111–120 (2008)
DOI: 10.1002/mpr

References

Abou-Sinna, R., & Luebbers, S. (2012). Validity of assessing people experiencing mental illness who have offended using the Camberwell Assessment of Need – Forensic and the Health of the Nation Outcome Scales – Secure. *International Journal of Mental Health Nursing, 21*, 462–470. https://doi.org/10.1111/j.1447-0349-2122.00811.x

Adams, J., Thomas, S.D.M., Mackinnon, T., & Eggleton, D. (2018). The risks, needs and stages of recovery of a complete forensic patient cohort in an Australian state. *BMC Psychiatry, 18*, 35. https://doi.org/10.1186/s12888-017-1584-8

Adams, J., Thomas, S.D.M., Mackinnon, T., & Eggleton, D. (2019). How secure are the secure psychiatric units in New South Wales? *Australasian Psychiatry, 27*, 32–35. https://doi.org/10.1177/1039856218804334

Barnao, M., & Ward, T. (2015). Sailing uncharted seas without a compass: A review of interventions in forensic mental health. *Aggression and Violent Behavior, 22*, 77–86. https://doi.org/10.1016/j.avb.2015.04.009

Buchanan, A., & Wootton, L. (2002). *Care of the Mentally Disordered Offender in the Community.* Oxford: Oxford University Press.

Castelletti, L., Lasavlia, A., Molinari, E., Thomas, S.D.M., Straticò, E., & Bonetto, C. (2014). A standardised tool for assessing needs in forensic psychiatric populations: Clinical validation of the Italian CANFOR, staff version. *Epidemiology and Psychiatric Services, 24*, 274–281. https://doi.org/10.1017/S2045796014000602

Chambers, J.C., Yiend, J., Barrett, B., Burns, T., Doll, H., Fazel, S., Jenkinson, C., Kaur, A., Knapp, M., Plugge, E., Sutton, L., & Fitzpatrick, R. (2009). Outcome measures used in forensic mental health research: A structured review. *Criminal Behaviour and Mental Health, 19*, 9–27. https://doi.org/10.1002/cbm.724

Chiswick, D. (1992). What mentally ill offenders need. *British Medical Journal, 304*, 267–268.

Davoren, M., O'Dwyer, S., Abidin, Z., Naughton, L., Gibbons, O., Doyle, E., McDonnell, K., Monks, S., & Kennedy, H.G. (2012). Prospective in-patient cohort study of moves between levels of therapeutic security: The DUNDRUM-1 triage security, DUNDRUM-3 programme completion and DUNDRUM-4 recovery scales and the HCR-20. *BMC Psychiatry, 12*, 80. https://doi.org/10.1186/1471-244X-12-80

Department of Health (1991). *The Care Programme Approach for People with a Mental Illness Referred to Specialist Mental Health Services.* London: Department of Health.

Department of Health (1999). *The National Service Framework for Mental Health.* London: Department of Health.

Department of Health / Home Office (1992). *Review of the Health and Social Services for Mentally Disordered Offenders and Others Requiring Similar Services. Final Summary Report (Cmnd 2088).* London: Her Majesty's Stationery Office.

Di Lorito, C., Völlm, B., & Denning, T. (2019). The characteristics and needs of older forensic psychiatric patients: A cross-sectional study in secure units within one UK regional service. *Journal of Forensic Psychiatry and Psychology, 30*, 975–992. https://doi.org/10.1080/14789949.2019.1659390

Dickens, G., Sugarman, P., & Walker, L. (2007). HoNOS-secure: A reliable outcome measure for users of secure and forensic mental health. *Journal of Forensic Psychiatry & Psychology, 18*, 507–514. https://doi.org/10.1080/14789940701492279

Dolan, M., Thomas, S.D., Thomas, S.L., & Thornicroft, G. (2005). The needs of males detained under the legal category of 'psychopathic disorder' in high security: Implications for policy and service development. *Journal of Forensic Psychiatry & Psychology, 16*, 523–537. https://doi.org/10.1080/14789940500097840

Douglas, K.S., Hart, S.D., Webster, C.D., & Belfrage, H. (2013). *HCR-20V3: Assessing Risk of Violence – User Guide.* Burnaby: Mental Health, Law, and Policy Institute, Simon Fraser University.

Hartwell, S. (2004). Triple stigma: Persons with mental illness and substance abuse problems in the criminal justice system. *Criminal Justice Policy Review, 15*, 84–99. https://doi.org/10.1177/0887403403255064

Harty, M.A., Jarrett, M., Thornicroft, G., & Shaw, J. (2012). Unmet needs of male prisoners under the care of prison mental health inreach services. *Journal of Forensic Psychiatry & Psychology, 23*, 285–296. https://doi.org/10.1080/14789949.2012.690101

Harty, M.A., Shaw, J., Thomas, S., Dolan, M., Davies, L., Thornicroft, G., Carlisle, J., Moreno, M., Leese, M., Appleby, L., & Jones, P. (2004). The security, clinical and social needs of patients in high security psychiatric hospitals in England. *Journal of Forensic Psychiatry & Psychology, 15*, 208–221. https://doi.org/10.1080/14789940410001703967

Home Office / Department of Health and Social Security (1975). *Report of the Committee on Mentally Abnormal Offenders (The Butler Report) (Cmnd 6244).* London: Her Majesty's Stationery Office.

Howard, L., Hunt, K., Slade, M., O'Keane, V., & Seneviratne, T. (2008). *CAN-M: Camberwell Assessment of Need for Mothers*. London: RC Psych Publications.

Isweran, M.S., & Bardsley, E.M. (1987). Secure facilities for mentally impaired patients. *Bulletin of the Royal College of Psychiatrists*, 11, 52–54.

Johnson, S., Thornicroft, G., Phelan, M. & Slade, M. (1996). Assessing needs for mental health services. In G. Thornicroft & M. Tansella (eds.), *Mental Health Outcome Measures*, pp. 217–226. New York: Springer.

Kennedy, H.G., O'Neill, C., Flynn, G., & Gill, P. (2010). *The Dundrum Toolkit: Dangerousness, Understanding, Recovery and Urgency Manual – The Dundrum Quartet*. Dublin: Trinity College Dublin.

Keulen-de Vos, M., & Schepers, K. (2016). Needs assessment in forensic patients: A review of instrument suites. *International Journal of Forensic Mental Health*, 15, 283–300. https://doi.org/10.1080/14999-13.2016.1152614

Livingston, J.D., Chu, K., Milne, T., & Brink, J. (2015). Probationers mandated to receive forensic mental health services in Canada: Risks/needs, service delivery, and intermediate outcomes. *Psychology, Public Policy, and Law*, 21, 72–84. https://doi.org/10.1037/law0000031

Livingston, J.D., Rossiter, K.R., & Verdun-Jones, S.N. (2011). 'Forensic' labelling: An empirical assessment of its effects on self-stigma for people with severe mental illness. *Psychiatry Research*, 188, 115–122. https://doi.org/10.1016/j.psychres.2011.01.018

Long, C., Webster, P., Waine, J., Motala, J., & Hollin, C.R. (2008). Usefulness of the CANFOR-S for measuring needs among mentally disordered offenders resident in medium or low secure hospital services in the UK: A pilot evaluation. *Criminal Behaviour and Mental Health*, 18, 39–48. https://doi.org/10.1002/cbm.676

NHS Management Executive (1990). *Services for Mentally Disordered Offenders and Difficult to Manage Patients (EL90/190)*. London: Department of Health.

Phelan, M., Slade, M., Thornicroft, G., Dunn, G., Holloway, F., Wykes, T., Strathdee, G., Loftus, L., McCrone, P., & Hayward, P. (1995). The Camberwell Assessment of Need: The validity and reliability of an instrument to assess the needs of the seriously mentally ill. *British Journal of Psychiatry*, 167, 589–595. https://doi.org/10.1192/bjp.167.5.589

Reynolds, T., Thornicroft, G., Abas, M., Woods, B., Hoe, J., Leese, M., & Orrell, M. (2000). Camberwell Assessment of Need for the Elderly (CANE): Development, validity and reliability. *British Journal of Psychiatry*, 176, 444–452. https://doi.org/10.1192/bjp.176.5.444

Romeo, G.E., Rubio, L.G., Guerre, S.O., Ramos Miravet, M. J., Caceres, A.G., & Thomas, S.D.M. (2010). Clinical validation of the CANFOR scale (Camberwell Assessment of Need – Forensic Version) for the needs assessment of people with mental health problems in the forensic services. *Actas Espanolas Psiquiatria*, 38, 129–137.

Royal College of Psychiatrists (1980). *Secure Facilities for Psychiatric Patients: A Comprehensive Policy*. London: Royal College of Psychiatrists.

Salvador-Carulla, L. (1996). Assessment instruments in psychiatry: description and psychometric properties. In G. Thornicroft & M. Tansella (eds.), *Mental Health Outcome Measures*. New York: Springer.

Segal, A., Daffern, M., Thomas, S., & Ferguson, M. (2010). Needs and risks of patients in a state-wide inpatient forensic mental health population. *International Journal of Mental Health Nursing* 19, 223–230. https://doi.org/10.1111/j.1447-0349.2010.00665.x

Semrau, M., van Ommeren, M., Blagescu, M., Griekspoor, A., Howard, L.M., Jordans, M., Melpp, H., Marini, A., Pedersen, J., Pilotte, I., Slade, M., & Thornicroft, G. (2012). The development and psychometric properties of the Humanitarian Emergency Settings Perceived Needs (HESPER) scale. *American Journal of Public Health*, 102, e55-63. https://doi.org/10.2105/AJPH.2012.300720

Shaw, J. (2002). Needs assessment for mentally disordered offenders is different. *Journal of Forensic Psychiatry*, 13, 14–17. https://doi.org/10.1080/09585180210123249

Shepherd, S.M., Ogloff, J.R.P., & Thomas, S.D.M. (2016). Are Australian prisons meeting the needs of Indigenous offenders? *Health & Justice*, 4, 13 (2016). https://doi.org/10.1186/s40352-016-0045-7

Shinkfield, G., & Ogloff, J. (2014). A review and analysis of routine outcome measures for forensic mental health services. *International Journal of Forensic Mental Health*, 13, 252–271. https://doi.org/10.1080/14999013.2014.939788

Shinkfield, G., & Ogloff, J. (2015). Use and interpretation of routine outcome measures in forensic mental health. *International Journal of Mental Health Nursing*, 24, 11–18. https://doi.org/10.1111/inm.12092

Slade, M., Phelan, M., Thornicroft, G., & Parkman, S. (1996). The Camberwell Assessment of Need (CAN): Comparison of assessments by staff and patients of the needs of the severely mentally ill. *Social Psychiatry and Psychiatric Epidemiology*, 31, 109–113. https://doi.org/10.1007/bf00785756

Slade, M., Phelan, M., & Thornicroft, G. (1998). A comparison of needs assessed by staff and an epidemiologically representative sample of patients with psychosis. *Psychological Medicine*, 28, 543–550. https://doi.org/10.1017/s0033291798006564

Slade, M., Thornicroft, G., Loftus, L., Phelan, M., & Wykes, T. (1999). *CAN: The Camberwell Assessment of Need*. London: Gaskell.

Slade, M., & Thornicroft, G. (2020). *Camberwell Assessment of Need (CAN)*, 2nd ed. Cambridge: Cambridge University Press.

Stevens, A., & Gabbay, J. (1991). Needs assessment needs assessment. *Health Trends*, 23, 20–23.

Talina, M., Cardoso, A., Aguiar, P., Caldas de Almeida, J., & Xavier, M. (2012). How different are the needs for care between forensic and civil psychiatric service users? *European Psychiatry*. https://doi.org/10.1016/S0924-9338(12)74848-4

Talina, M., Thomas, S., Cardosa, A., Aguiar, P., Caldas de Almeida, J.M., & Xavier, M. (2013). CANFOR Portuguese version: validation study. *BMC Psychiatry*, *13*, 157. https://doi.org/10.1186/1471-244X-13-157

Thomas, S.D., Dolan, M., Johnston, S., Middleton, H., Harty, M.A., Carlisle, J., Thornicroft, G., Appleby, L., & Jones, P. (2004). Defining the needs of patients with intellectual disabilities in the high security psychiatric hospitals in England. *Journal of Intellectual Disability Research*, *48*, 603–610. https://doi.org/10.1111/j.1365-2788.2004.00629.x

Thomas, S.D.M., Dolan, M., Shaw, J., Thomas, S., Thornicroft, S., Thornicroft, G., & Leese, M. (2005). Redeveloping secure psychiatric services for women. *Medicine, Science and the Law*, *45*, 331–339. https://doi.org/10.1258/rsmmsl.45.4.331

Thomas, S., Dolan, M., & Thornicroft, G. (2004). Re-visiting the need for High Security Psychiatric Hospitals in England. *Journal of Forensic Psychiatry & Psychology*, *15*, 197–207. https://doi.org/10.1080/1478990410001703976

Thomas, S., Harty, M.A., Parrott, J., McCrone, P., Slade, M., & Thornicroft, G. (2003). *CANFOR: Camberwell Assessment of Need – Forensic Version*. London: Gaskell.

Thomas, D., Leese, M., Dolan, M., Harty, M.A., Shaw, J., Middleton, H., Davies, L., Thornicroft, G., & Appleby, L. (2004). The individual needs of patients in high secure psychiatric hospitals in England. *Journal of Forensic Psychiatry & Psychology*, *15*, 222–243. https://doi.org/10.1080/14789940410001702283

Thomas, S., McCrone, P., & Fahy, T. (2009). How do psychiatric patient on prison healthcare centres differ from inpatients in secure psychiatric inpatient units? *Psychology, Crime & Law*, *15*, 729–742. https://doi.org/10.1080/10683160802516365

Thomas, S.D.M., Slade, M., McCrone, P., Harty, M.A., Parrott, J., Thornicroft, G., & Leese, M. (2008). The reliability and validity of the forensic Camberwell Assessment of Need (CANFOR): A needs assessment for forensic mental health service users. *International Journal of Methods in Psychiatric Research*, *17*, 111–120. https://doi.org/10.1002/mpr.235

Working Party on Security in NHS Hospitals (1974). *Revised Report (Glancy Report)*. London: Department of Health and Social Security.

Xenitidis, K., Thornicroft, G., Leese, M., Slade, M., Fotiadou, M., Philp, H., Sayer, J., Harris, E., McGee, D., & Murphy, D.G.M. (2000). Reliability and validity of CANDID – a needs assessment instrument for adults with learning disabilities and mental health problems. *British Journal of Psychiatry*, *176*, 473–478. https://doi.org/10.1192/bjp.176.5.473

Index